MENTAL HEALTH IN LATE MEDIAEVAL ENGLAND

*For Micha.
I know you would have read it.*

MENTAL HEALTH IN LATE MEDIAEVAL ENGLAND

A SURPRISING HISTORY OF MENTAL ILLNESS AND ITS TREATMENT IN SOCIETY

MICHÈLE SCHINDLER

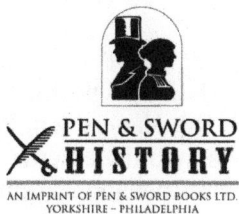

PEN & SWORD
HISTORY
AN IMPRINT OF PEN & SWORD BOOKS LTD.
YORKSHIRE – PHILADELPHIA

First published in Great Britain in 2025 by
PEN AND SWORD HISTORY
An imprint of
Pen & Sword Books Ltd
Yorkshire – Philadelphia

Copyright © Michèle Schindler, 2025

ISBN 978 1 39909 244 9

The right of Michèle Schindler to be identified as Author of this work has been asserted by her in accordance with the Copyright, Designs and Patents Act 1988.

A CIP catalogue record for this book is available from the British Library.

All rights reserved. No part of this book may be reproduced, transmitted, downloaded, decompiled or reverse engineered in any form or by any means, electronic or mechanical including photocopying, recording or by any information storage and retrieval system, without permission from the Publisher in writing. No part of this book may be used or reproduced in any manner for the purpose of training artificial intelligence technologies or systems.

Typeset in Times New Roman 11.5/14 by
SJmagic DESIGN SERVICES, India.
Printed and bound in the UK by CPI Group (UK) Ltd.

The Publisher's authorised representative in the EU for product safety is Authorised Rep Compliance Ltd., Ground Floor, 71 Lower Baggot Street, Dublin D02 P593, Ireland.
www.arccompliance.com

For a complete list of Pen & Sword titles please contact
PEN & SWORD BOOKS LIMITED
George House, Units 12 & 13, Beevor Street, Off Pontefract Road, Barnsley, South Yorkshire, S71 1HN, England
E-mail: enquiries@pen-and-sword.co.uk
Website: www.pen-and-sword.co.uk

or
PEN AND SWORD BOOKS
1950 Lawrence Rd, Havertown, PA 19083, USA
E-mail: uspen-and-sword@casematepublishers.com
Website: www.penandswordbooks.com

Contents

Preface vi
Introduction viii

Chapter 1 Famous cases 1
                1.1. Unspecified mental health issues 1
                1.2. Suicide 19
Chapter 2 Treatments for mental illnesses 32
                2.1. General treatments 32
                2.2. Religious treatments 48
                2.3. Suspected causes and how they affected
                      treatments 54
Chapter 3 Societal reaction 61
                3.1. Legal ramifications of mental illness 103
                3.2. Accusations of insanity and weird behaviour 109
                3.3. Modern prejudices 120
Chapter 4 Religion and mental illness 124
Chapter 5 Mental health and mental illness in mediaeval
                literature 152

Appendices 165
Endnotes 188

Preface

Mental health and mental illnesses are broad subjects. Despite a recent surge in interest in them, they have not yet been fully understood. Even the definition of what mental health is and what constitutes a mental illness differs, depending on the exact question and who is doing the asking.

It is no surprise, then, that mental health and mental illnesses throughout history is an equally difficult subject. Given the challenges of discussing these subjects even under a contemporary lens, it is unsurprising that mental health and mental illnesses in the Middle Ages are subjects that are very under-explored. This book is an attempt to bridge this gap, at least to an extent, by looking at famous cases of mental illnesses in mediaeval Europe and exploring the way mental health and mental illnesses were understood at the time.

Since these subjects are too expansive for a single book if it attempted to cover all of mediaeval Europe, the focus will lie on the late Middle Ages and early Renaissance (twelfth to sixteenth century) in England, with only passing references to other countries such as France and Spain, for comparison.

Though there were different understandings of what mental health and mental illness even were during the Middle Ages, which is explored in this book, the modern definition of mental illness which this book is using as a basis, has been summed up with the help of the book *Cry of Pain: Understanding Suicide and the Suicidal Mind* by Professor Mark Williams.[1]

'Mental illness in the modern day is loosely defined as a period (acute or chronic) in which a person experiences a range of psychopathological symptoms. These range from depression, anxiety and problems with mood regulation through to hearing voices (hallucinations), delusions, and psychosis. In the modern-day mental illness is often identified through medical texts grounded in research, the DSM-V and ICD-10 for example and is treated via medical treatments (e.g. medication) and psychological therapies.'

This definition, and the details following from it,[2] will be the framework with which the cases of mediaeval mental illness will be examined, so they can be understood in modern terms.

Introduction

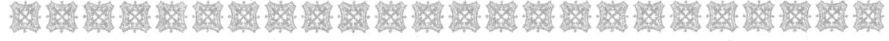

In his book *The Reign of Henry VI: The Exercise of Royal Authority*, the historian, Ralph Alan Griffiths, stated that when Henry VI 'suffered a severe mental collapse'[3] in the summer of 1453, 'there was no doctor and no known medicine that could cure him'. He goes on to say that this illness meant that his very dynasty was in danger, as '[t]he Lancastrian hold on the throne was never so precarious as it was in 1453'.[4]

This book is a well-researched, excellent and very scholarly one, but by saying this and making a judgement not only on Henry VI's policies but also on late mediaeval mental health care, it rests on the often-repeated assumptions of the lack of understanding of mental health and mental illnesses at the time. It is a judgement that has been echoed for centuries. Similar views can be found in many newer books.

Though leaps and bounds have been made in mental health care in the late twentieth and early twenty-first centuries, much stigma is still attached to many mental health problems. Such stigmas sadly often colour the description of how illnesses of that sort were treated in late mediaeval England as much as the stigmas of the time obscure our understanding of the issues. To try and reach the most complete picture possible of how mental health was regarded, treated and considered in late mediaeval England, there need not only be an understanding of how primary sources treated it, but also how historians in later centuries did when working with those sources.

Only when taking all this into account can we truly begin to understand these issues.

Chapter 1

Famous cases

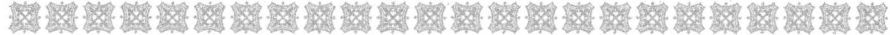

1.1. Unspecified mental health issues

There is more information than is often thought about mental health, mental illness and treatment of such in late mediaeval and early modern Europe. It was long thought to be a subject that was mostly hushed up at the time, which has not generated much interest in the centuries afterwards and has been compared to modern day treatments without much context.[5] However, it is a misconception that mental illness was not of much interest in late mediaeval England. In fact, there are several instances of important men and women being recorded to have mental health issues, and of those being recorded without any distaste, but instead very similarly to how physical illnesses were recorded.

What this means, of course, is that we have a wealth of information about mental health and mental illnesses in late mediaeval England, but the information is sadly unspecific. Occasionally, symptoms were described,[6] but more often than not, euphemisms were used.[7] This was common in the way any illness was recorded in sources in the fourteenth and fifteenth century, with even physicians' bills and records not giving any specific names for illnesses.[8] Often those bills only recorded the ingredients for a medicine, without stating its use. Even when the use is recorded, it is usually vague, such as 'a preciose water for all maner of poison and namely for pestilence for as philosophers seyn it is impossibull that any man shuld dcy of poison and of pestilence who so usith to drynk of that water'. Medical research about that time has to rely on guesswork because of this reason. This makes the research harder, but it also gives the researcher the possibility of working out how several illnesses, today given exact names, were seen at the time — which symptoms were considered the most important, which conclusions were drawn from it, as well as which treatments were offered.

The most famous person in mediaeval England with mental health issues is Henry VI, the man who became king at the age of only 9 months in August 1421 and is in fact best known for growing up mentally unwell. 'The baby king who grew up an imbecile'[9] as he was called by historian K.B. McFarlane,[10] has been a subject of much derision by historians since his death, with his mental illness often making him a subject of ridicule. However, this was not the case during his own lifetime, not even after he had been usurped and his usurper, the first Yorkist king, Edward IV, had a vested interest in making him unsuitable to rule. While Yorkist propaganda naturally made use of Henry's mental illness,[11] it did not actually use it to ridicule him or present him as a bad person because of it.

This is in stark contrast to what is often believed about the time. The historian, Bertram Wolffe, famously spoke about Henry VI rarely making 'little consistent effort'[12] to succeed as a king and connected his failings, such as supposedly undue generosity, to his 'madness'.[13] In fact, in his biography of the unlucky king, Wolffe goes so far to imply it was lucky Henry went mad. His reasoning was that Henry thus could not rule for long periods of time, because 'he was both an incompetent and a partisan king',[14] implying that his madness both made him a bad king and was used against him, a judgement that has often been repeated. Biographers more sympathetic to Henry have stressed his kind nature[15] but have often taken his mental illness either as a sign of him being unable to cope with being king, or else making him unable to be king.[16] Though rarely spelled out, the implication is usually that his contemporaries thought similarly.[17] However, primary sources do not at all support this.

In fact, many primary sources about Henry VI's illness are fairly matter of fact. Though there was some gossip about him being 'mad', and several people were punished for it,[18] none of his political opponents used his mental illness to attack him. The illness was described in the same kind of terms used for physical illnesses, but again, there was no name attached to the symptoms he showed. This has made it easy for researchers to assume he had any number of mental illnesses we have a name for today, but that were not known under such a name at the time. Personality disorder, schizophrenia and paranoia have been only some of the illnesses that have been suggested,[19] all with the use of primary sources, all interpreting the symptoms these sources record.

The fact that Henry VI's maternal grandfather, King Charles VI of France, is also known to have suffered from a mental illness has even given rise to the theory that Henry inherited this illness from him, though Henry VI's most recent biographer, Lauren Johnson, has pointed out that the symptoms of their illnesses do not resemble each other at all.[20] While Charles VI was recorded to have had spells during which he believed he was being followed by unseen assassins, Henry never showed any signs of suffering from such delusions. Instead, the primary sources speak of him being unable to react to his surroundings at all and of being very childlike in manner.[21] The occasional bouts of cruelty, which did not appear to suit his character, were not, by contemporaries, attributed to his illness.[22] Instead, usually those close to Henry were blamed for such actions, though sometimes, the evidence does not bear this out.[23] Of course, it was hardly unusual for a mediaeval king to occasionally be cruel, and in itself this is not a sign of mental illness, but it was noted to be in stark contrast to Henry's usual personality, and to usually be followed by strong regret.[24] That this was not considered to be part of his mental illness is therefore interesting.

Another sign of mental instability reported in Henry was what would today be called religious mania[25] which was seen as unusual and slightly alarming in Henry's own time,[26] enough so to be recorded and in fact counted as a symptom of his illness.

However, the strange treatment of Henry VI and his illness is not a singular case, even if it is the most famous one, as well as the most talked about. There are several other cases which also received quite a bit of attention at the time, some of them almost or completely contemporary to Henry VI.

One such case is that of William Beaumont, Viscount Beaumont, who was born in 1438. Unlike Henry, his mental illness has never been considered genetic, neither contemporarily nor later, but seen as the result of his bad experiences during the Wars of the Roses. Because of that, William's case is also a very interesting one, as it illustrates the understanding of how circumstances could influence mental health.

With our modern understanding of mental health, it is definitely understandable that William suffered from the consequences of what he experienced during the Wars of the Roses. Remarked upon even in contemporary sources to be a peace-loving man, he was forced into the conflict between Lancastrian forces and Yorkist forces through his father's involvement in them. Unlike his son, John Beaumont, Viscount Beaumont, was a warlike man[27] whose closeness to Queen Margaret, Henry VI's wife, made him a perfect candidate to fight in the conflicts. He was noted to do so, and it was that which eventually killed him when he fell at the Battle of Northampton on 10 July 1460.[28] His death left William in a position of having to step into his father's shoes as one of the queen's most important men, at the age of 22. William was noted to be a peaceful man and his contemporary, the chronicler Robert Bale, quoted him as saying that he was content with 'let[ting] each man place his feet in the soil as the good lord intended'[29] — in other words, letting each man do as he decided to do. As such, he implied he had no quarrel with anyone supporting another candidate as king as he did, but due to his father's decisions in the civil war, he had to fight. He was involved in several battles, including the Battle of Towton, which has since been called the biggest battle to ever take place on English soil, with an estimate being that 20,000 people died in it. William's side lost, and the victorious new king, Edward IV, arrested him. Unlike most of his fellow fighters, William was not released after several months but seemed doomed to stay in prison indefinitely.

He prevented that by escaping after around eight months in prison, making his way to exile in France, where Henry VI's queen, Margaret of Anjou, was also staying. He did not get to see his home again for nine years, during which time his younger sister and his oldest nephew died. It is possible he re-connected with his sister's younger children when he returned to England for a short while during the Lancastrian readeption in late 1470 and early 1471, but if so, it was a short-lived pleasure. After around six months, he once more had to take part in several battles, his side lost once more, and he once more had to leave for exile.

Interestingly, despite his noted peaceful nature, his reaction was a violent one. Together with his friend and fellow fighter, John de Vere, Earl of Oxford, he engaged in piracy to try and cause as much trouble as he could for Edward IV, and perhaps also facilitate his overthrow. This, however, ended in disaster for him once again. After being besieged at St Michael's Mount, he was eventually forced to surrender; he and John were imprisoned by Edward IV's men. They stayed in prison at Hammes Castle, which is near Calais, for nearly twelve years, until they were finally able to escape in 1484.

A year later, William finally got his chance to return to England for good, by once more taking part in a battle — the Battle of Bosworth Field. However, any fond hopes he had to reunite with his second oldest nephew, his only family member then still alive whom he would have been able to remember from his time as a young man, were dashed. His nephew, Francis, Viscount Lovell, the closest friend of King Richard III who was killed at the Battle of Bosworth Field, was not ready to accept his friend's usurper. Instead, Viscount Lovell began several assassination attempts and two rebellions against the newly crowned king, Henry VII.

Evidence suggests his nephew's attitude was the tipping point for William and was what triggered his mental illness. From 1486 onwards, he was noted to act strange and erratic and in November 1487, his mental illness, whatever it was, had become so bad that he was considered unsuitable to take care of his own lands. The matter was put to parliament and considered, with the result that his lands and possessions were given to William's friend, John de Vere, Earl of Oxford, to manage in William's best interest. The reasoning given for this is as interesting as the decision in itself:

> 'Since that restoration our said sovereign lord has become convinced that the same viscount does not have the gravity and discretion to rule and keep himself or his said livelihood, but since that time has alienated, wasted, spoiled and put away a great part of it most unwisely, to the disinheritance of him and his heirs, and in all likelihood, should he have his liberty, he would hereafter deal with what is left in the same way.
>
> In consideration of which, and since our said sovereign lord is bound to make provision for such persons as have inheritance and lack the gravity and discretion to rule and keep the same without alienation or the disinheritance of their heirs, by the advice of the lords spiritual and temporal and the commons assembled in this present parliament, and by authority of the same, be it ordained, decreed and enacted

that our sovereign lord the king, or such as his grace shall depute, shall have the rule, disposition and guidance of all the livelihood and inheritance to which the said viscount was restored by the act of restitution made for him in the parliament held in the first year of the reign of our said sovereign lord, during the life of the same viscount, to the honour, maintenance and profit of the said viscount; and that the same viscount, during that time, shall have no authority or power to give or grant any part of it to any person without the assent or agreement of our said sovereign lord, while the said viscount is in the custody of our said sovereign lord, or the assent and agreement of such as his grace shall depute to have the rule of the said livelihood and inheritance; saving to all the king's liege people, other than the said viscount, such right, title and lawful interest as they have in or to any of the things stated.'[30]

Obviously, whatever William suffered from, it made him behave rather erratically and in such a way that he was not thought to be able to act in his own interest, as well as anyone else's. Even so, the tone of the parliamentary decision is notably lacking in any judgement about this. In comparison to similar decisions from the 1800s or even the early 1900s, it could almost be called compassionate. William's symptoms are described in a dry and precise-sounding way, and though the negative effects his behaviour had on him and others were mentioned, there were no personal attacks included.

The decision itself also shows a remarkable lack of punishment for William, running contrary to what is still believed to have been the custom in late mediaeval England, and how it was described in later centuries.[31] First and foremost, it was what was considered to be best for William in his situation. The king did not try in any way to profit from William's lands and possessions himself or enact something that could have been harmful to him. Instead, by giving these lands to William's friend of well over a decade, it was made sure that it was in the hands of someone who could be trusted to keep his wellbeing in mind, rather than exploit the new possessions he had been given.

It could be argued, of course, that William, much like Henry VI, was a special case, hardly a normal one. He had known his king, Henry VII, since Henry had been a teenager, and his friend the Earl of Oxford was in fact known to be close to the king. Therefore, it could be that the kindness to William was either only due to his long acquaintance with the king, or else simply coincidental, a happy but unintended side effect of Henry wanting to reward one of his closest men. John de Vere, Earl of Oxford, was claimed by many to have been instrumental in winning the Battle of Bosworth Field and therefore also his kingship for Henry VII. It would make sense, therefore, if Henry wished to reward him. However, even if this was the case, and the king's kindness is not revealing of general attitudes towards mental illness, the general treatment of William certainly is. Even if Henry VII was motivated by selfish reasons, not compassion or kindness, which is unknowable, he was not the one to write the parliamentary rolls. There would have been no point for those who did to use non-discriminatory language if such language were common and accepted in such cases otherwise. The matter-of-fact way it was treated even in such official documents definitely indicates that while 'acceptance' is too strong a word to choose, there was certainly some compassion towards those who suffered from mental health issues.

There is a suggestion that William's illness was what we today would call bipolar disorder.[32] Certainly, this would make sense of what little we know from the parliament rolls; overspending and making frivolous purchases and even presents, while at other times being dejected and depressed, are both very typical symptoms of this illness.[33] However, there is no saying if there were perhaps other symptoms as well, which were not considered relevant to his being thought to be unsuitable to take care of his own possessions, and which might open up another possibility of mental illness.

However, the exact nature of his illness is not very relevant, as it was not considered to be so at the time. Far more interesting is the way it was viewed. Interestingly, even in 1487, when William's mental illness was in its infancy, the mention of it in the parliamentary rolls did not anticipate his recovery. Instead, it was assumed that he would never be well enough to take care of his own lands again. This could, once more, be seen more as a political move than any knowledge of mental illnesses at the time. It could be problematic for the king to strip one his closest and most important supporters of a fairly substantial amount of lands and possessions he had granted him. On the other hand, holding lands for someone else was usually not a grant designed to last — it was something usually connected with wardships, which would end once the ward came of age. Moreover, with the Earl of Oxford being William Beaumont's friend, it might not have been too much of a problem for anyone involved if William recovered. Therefore, the fact that no recovery was expected might have been a genuine expectation, rather than a political one.

In any case, it was the correct assumption. Not only did William not recover, over time his illness became worse. By 1495, it had become so bad that the matter was taken to parliament again because he was considered unable to take care of himself. Once more, the language of the decision reached is worth quoting in full:

> 'Where in the parliament held at Westminster on 9 November in the third year of the reign of our sovereign lord the king [1487], it was ordained, decreed and enacted, for various good considerations contained in the said act, that our said sovereign lord or such as his grace should depute should have the rule, disposition and guidance of all the livelihood and inheritance of William, Viscount Beaumont, to which the said viscount was restored by an act of restitution made for him in the parliament held at Westminster in the first year of our said sovereign lord's reign [1485], during the life of the said viscount; and that the said viscount during that time should have no authority to give or grant any part of it to any person without the assent and agreement of our said sovereign lord or the assent and agreement of such as his grace should depute, while the said viscount was in the keeping of our said sovereign lord, or of such as his grace should depute to have the rule of the said livelihood or inheritance; in which act it was not clear what form the king's licence should take in that matter, or how the person of the said viscount should be kept, ordered, guided and conducted, but it was left open, as a result of which things might be done which were not to the king's honour, or to the worship of this land, considering he is a person descended of the noble blood of this land.
>
> For which reason it is ordained, enacted and decreed by authority of this present parliament that the king our sovereign lord, or such as he has or shall depute and assign, shall take

and have the conduct, rule, keeping and governance, during the life of the [col. b] said viscount, of the person of the said viscount as well as of his said livelihood and inheritance, to be applied to the sustenance and maintenance of the said viscount as well as to the payment of his debts and otherwise, as shall be thought necessary and desirable by the king our sovereign lord, and by such as he has or shall depute and assign in that matter; and that the said viscount shall have no authority or power to give, grant, charge or alienate any part of his said livelihood or inheritance during his said life without the king's licence under his great seal; and if any alienation, gift, grant or charge has been made by him without obtaining the king's licence under his great seal in that matter since the said act was made in the said third year of his reign, except presentations to churches, chapels and chantries, then that alienation, gift, grant or charge shall stand and be entirely void and of no effect, except for those before excepted: and that no person shall hereafter be vexed or hurt by the said viscount, his executors or any other person claiming to his use any part of the said livelihood or inheritance, for any occupation or intervention, by reason of this act or since the said act made in the said third year of the king our sovereign lord's reign.'[34]

Here, for the first time, we see some embarrassment about William being inflicted with a mental illness, or rather, the possibility of embarrassment. The fear that his behaviour had become so bad it could be an embarrassment for the king definitely speaks to there being a stigma attached to William's illness, but of course, this could be overstated. Since the parliamentary entry does not give any details as to what this behaviour was like, it could be that it was genuinely harmful behaviour, either to William or someone else physically, or to the king's position.

If so, it would be only natural to want to stop any such behaviour. Moreover, it was not all that easy to declare someone unable to take care of himself, not even at the time, as will be discussed below. Therefore, a reason as to why the decision was taken had to be included.

It is also notable that despite this, the language is once more dry, precise and not at all in any way inflammatory. If anything, the language sounds compassionate, and in this case, the decision as to whose ward he was to become was also well considered.

As mentioned above, the decision to grant William's possessions to his long-time friend, the Earl of Oxford, might very well have been a political one, as it was one that made one of the king's closest supporters richer. However, the decision of who was to take care of his person was not. If anything, the Earl of Oxford having to take care of William was fiscally disadvantageous for him. Previously, his holding of William's lands and possessions came with few strings attached. As he was not indifferent to William, he must have had an interest in taking good care of him, but there was nothing actually requiring him to do so. Apart from a need to leave enough money for William to be able to keep up his standard of living, he was free to do with his money whatever he pleased. Once he had custody of William's person, though, rather than just his lands, a lot of the income generated by the Beaumont lands would have had to have been spent on William's upkeep.

However, while William's case appears to have been discussed at the time, as was only natural, either nobody thought that having to take care of him was a burden for the Earl of Oxford, or nobody wrote down such thoughts. Again, rather than repulsion, those who knew of the case appear to have reacted with understanding and compassion.

This counts for the king as well. Henry VII was usually not noted for his compassionate nature, though the extent of his tyranny has been exaggerated in recent years. There is no doubt, though, that even had he been inclined to, he could not allow any sort of doubt about his kingship, and any attack on it, to go unpunished. In the light of this, the fact that William had acted in some way to embarrass or potentially even harm Henry and was not punished, but treated with compassion, is quite notable.

There is no actual hint of what this behaviour was, only that it not only upset the king in some way but also was blatant enough that parliament agreed it was both upsetting as well as harmful to William himself if allowed to continue. One possibility is that he attempted to commit suicide. This would, of course, have been an attempt to commit a mortal sin. By mediaeval standards, this would have been the worst that could happen, not only for William himself but also for those around him. If he had succeeded, then by the ecclesiastical laws of the time, he would have been damned forever, with no chance at redemption. He would not have been allowed to be buried in hallowed ground, and he would have been a criminal. This would mean all his possessions would be forfeit to the crown, with his wife not inheriting anything.

This was not always followed, as will be seen later, but quite obviously, if William had attempted suicide, it would be considered important to keep him from trying again, not just for ecclesiastical reasons and secular laws, but also for his own sake. If he was truly bipolar, or rather exhibited symptoms of what would today be called bipolarity, then it might have been considered a good idea for him to be close to a man who was his friend. The reasons for this are clear: a friend would have been able to catch his more sombre moods before they could escalate and prevent the worst. However, there are two problems with this theory: for one, the person of John de Vere, Earl of Oxford himself. Though he was a staunch supporter of Henry VII, and a very matter-of-fact man, his own history of mental health problems[35] would have made him an unlikely carer for William if indeed he was suicidal.

The second problem with this theory is that William was taken care of in such a way that he never truly seemed to realise he was ill, or at least not that he was being taken care of in his friend's household because of it. This is certainly interesting, because upon being made Oxford's ward in 1495, he moved to the earl's favourite manor of Wivenhoe[36] and there is evidence he never left again until his death. It is unlikely that William, who we know was certainly coherent enough to think of making small legal grants at least occasionally, did not realise where he was. In 1488 he was witness to a bond[37] and in 1498, he made a grant of a book to his wife.[38] The latter especially suggests that he was unaware of any mental problems plaguing him at that moment, and suggests that he had moments of clarity. However, just those moments of clarity also suggest that he was equally unaware of what his situation actually was like. There is no evidence of him expressing surprise at it, or even wishing to clear up that he was 'sound of mind' at the moment of writing, rather than just treating it as a generic formula with which legal writings were to be prefaced, without having a personal significance.

This argues against William being suicidal at any point, as doubtlessly, when feeling well and not in the grips of such an impulse, he would be aware of having experienced it. This would suggest that his mental illness was such that he himself did not realise it. This is far from uncommon for a number of illnesses, bipolar disorder among them,[39] but does not usually include suicidal thoughts,[40] which by definition are hard to ignore.

Though we can make some deductions as to the nature of William's illness with such logic and by process of elimination, it is virtually impossible to make any reasonably accurate diagnosis after so long a time, with so little information as to the symptoms William suffered. What is known, though, is that William was not treated badly at all. In fact, as detailed above, he was obviously treated in such a way that he was not even aware anything was wrong at all. Though this was also in some ways influenced by his illness, as otherwise he would have grasped the significance of being made to live with his friend and having no control over his own lands and possessions, all was done to make him believe that he was in complete control of his own life. Unlike the dark thoughts often connected with pre-modern health care, such as confinement so as not to be socially visible and an embarrassment, or worries of being an outcast, ignored or even reviled by friends and family, there were no dark dungeons in which William was kept so as not to embarrass anyone, nor torturous treatments to startle him back to mental health. What seemed to be done was mostly in kindness, ensuring his stay in the gilded cage he was in and his illness that he was unable to escape from, was as comfortable and closely resembling normalcy as at all possible.

This illusion of normal appears to have been kept up by those around him until his death in 1507, by which time he had suffered from mental illness for twenty years. Not only did the Earl of Oxford try and keep things as routine as possible for him, so too did Oxford's wife Margaret and, significantly, William's wife, Elizabeth Scrope, as well as all the servants who were employed to take care of him.

William's illness appears to have become steadily worse, and in the last five years of his life, we know nothing of his treatments and actions at all. Possibly, by that time, he was unable to function at all anymore without outside help, much like Friedrich Nietzsche several centuries later,[41] but as his care was considered suitable and caused no problems, we cannot say. All we know is that when he died, the Earl of Oxford had a splendid tomb erected for him, with an effigy. There would have been absolutely no need for him to do that; it was far from common for any noble, and nobody would have blamed Oxford if he simply had a less expensive but still honourable burial and grave. That he did not shows it was a decision made for himself, wanting to honour William.

This high regard in which William was held is another point of interest and shows once more that mental illness was treated much more like today than is commonly thought, and was not something that made people instantly distance themselves from the sufferer. Not only did the Earl of Oxford hold William in high regard until his death, without thinking any less of him because he suffered from a mental illness, the same is true for William's wife. In fact, in some ways her case is much more telling, because she only married William in 1486 and unlike Oxford, would therefore not have known William without his mental illness.

Elizabeth Scrope, daughter of Sir Richard Scrope, came from a Yorkist family and had been married to William as a rapprochement between her family and the Lancastrian/Tudor cause in April 1486, when she was 18 years old and William was nearly 50. Such marriages happened often during this time, as the personal feelings of husband and wife towards one another were irrelevant. This particular match was obviously motivated by politics. Elizabeth therefore had no reason to feel particularly close to her husband, but despite this, we know that she came to care for him. In fact, when she made her will nearly thirty years after William's death, she named only him as her husband, instead of naming both him and her second husband, the Earl of Oxford, and requested to be laid to rest next to him.[42]

Obviously, she deeply cared for him. This, too, was not uncommon, not even in such matches which sound shocking to modern ears. In Elizabeth and William's case, it is certainly interesting, though. It was in the very year of their wedding that the first signs of William's mental illness were either noticed or recorded, but Elizabeth was not only not repulsed, but she came to love her husband. Again, this shows that the widespread picture of mental illness and its reception in the Middle Ages is incorrect, and that those who suffered from it were not automatically seen as repulsive.[43] In fact, William's whole case shows that this is not true: he was treated with kindness by the king, by his guardian, loved by his wife and held in high regard by friends. There is no negative comment about him recorded, no indication anyone thought any less of him because he suffered from an unspecified mental illness. Even the official language in parliament when the case was brought to their attention was dry and compassionate, rather than inflammatory and accusing.

In fact, for England there is quite a wealth of evidence for mentally ill people, especially nobles, and their treatment. One interesting case, happening when William was a child, and almost exactly at the same time as Henry VI's own mental illness first emerged, is that of George Neville, Lord Latimer. George was from a rich and wealthy family, with royal blood and thus fairly closely related to the king; he was either the third or the fifth son of Joan Beaufort and Ralph Neville, Earl of Westmorland.[44] The Neville family and their importance in fifteenth-century English politics have been amply recorded elsewhere, and what is important for this study is that they were well known, wealthy and influential. They had strengthened their own position in the fifteenth century by marrying into other important families, which passed on new titles to members of their family. George himself had done so, marrying Lady Elizabeth, daughter of Sir Richard Beauchamp and his first wife Elizabeth de Berkley, and becoming Lord Latimer after his uncle's death. There is very little known about his first fifty or so years of life, and all that there is suggests he was a quiet and conventional nobleman, who spent his time managing his and his wife's estates, having a number of children to whom he intended to eventually pass on his possessions. All the rest, we can only guess, but there is no suggestion whatsoever, much less any evidence, that he was in any way unconventional, considered to be strange or that anyone tried to challenge his hold on his lands. However, this does not have to mean anything, as it is obvious that we do not have all the evidence we would need to know everything about his life; undoubtedly parts of his life are lost to us.

As far as the sources we have suggest, George suddenly and unexpectedly became mentally so unwell that he was unable to have control of his own lands, and they were granted to his oldest brother Richard Neville, Earl of Salisbury, in consideration of this. There is no evidence of this being considered a punishment, of George being shrouded in shame and was therefore being punished by having his lands and possessions taken from him, and in fact, the language of the grant to the Earl of Salisbury suggests the opposite:

> 'Grant to Richard, earl of Salisbury, brother of George Neville, lord of Latimer, in consideration of the latter's love of the former, of the keeping of all lordships, manors, lands, offices, possessions, advowsons and hereditaments,

which pertain to the king by reason of the idiocy of the said George, to hold during the life of George.'[45]

The very fact that the grant mentioned that George's lands were given to the Earl of Salisbury because he loved his brother, rather than being kept in the king's hands, is quite telling as to how at least mentally ill noblemen were treated in England in the mid-fifteenth century. There was no recrimination and there was a degree of kindness, a wish to do what was best for the person stricken with the illness. To give the lands and possessions of the mentally ill man to his brother, explicitly due to his brother loving him, must have doubtlessly been intended to assure that George received only the best care. Moreover, there would certainly have been an element of making sure that in the event of him becoming better, his brother could allow him to have a say in the management of his lands.

It has sometimes been argued that the language suggesting kindness towards George was but a smokescreen, to hide the real intentions of punishing George for having a mental illness. However, there is no way this can be supported by any of the scant evidence that survives, and in fact, it does not really make a lot of sense. If mentally ill people were really treated with so much prejudice that there was a desire by the king and/or the nobles to punish them for it, then there would have been absolutely no need to hide it behind words which obviously suggested the very opposite. If there was no such prejudice, thus necessitating the use of such language as a smokescreen, there was also absolutely no reason to punish George for his mental illness. In other words, logic dictates that the grant was honest and that there was no backhandedness, no sly actions to strip George of his right, but simply an intention to do what was best for him in the face of his sudden 'idiocy'.

Sadly, there are no indications just what this 'idiocy' was, or when it started. Nor is there any indication what symptoms George had, how they were treated, how his life changed apart from him no longer having custody of his own lands or any other piece of information that could help us put together a more coherent picture of his life once he was declared an 'idiot'. Once more, we can only go by bits and pieces, by the evidence of absence of any sort of vitriol against him.

Probably because of the dearth of sources, several historians have tried to fill the gaps by making assumptions. In her work *The Nevills of Middleham: England's Most Powerful Family in the Wars of the Roses*, the author, Karen Clark, asserted that George had a mental breakdown in around 1440[46] but since she does not source this claim, it must be treated as pure guesswork. In John Burke's *A General and Heraldic Dictionary of the Peerages of England, Ireland, and Scotland, Extinct, Dormant, and in Abeyance* as well, the idea that George was already suffering from a mental illness as early as 1440 is presumed to have been very likely,[47] but again, since there are no sources given, this cannot be confirmed or denied. It is, in short, pure guesswork as well.

George's first forty to fifty years of life appear to have passed without him ever having any sort of mental illness, or at the very least, with him not showing symptoms that were so bad they were recorded anywhere. Only when he was nearly 50 did his mental illness either start or become so bad that it was considered unwise to let him control his own lands. Some have speculated that his mental illness was to do with his age. John Burke, for example, suggested that he suffered from a form of dementia.[48] Though, at the age of 50, George would be very young to be suffering from this disease, this is far from impossible; he might very well have suffered from early-onset dementia. However, there is nothing by way of evidence to support this, any more than there is any evidence to debunk it. Henry VI and his grandfather, Charles VI, had themselves only started suffering from mental illnesses when well into their adulthood. Evidence suggests George was another example.

It is, however, particularly notable that George was not actually connected with his mental illness in the public mind. We know this from several contemporary sources, most notably *Gregory's Chronicle*, written in the time between 1450 and 1470,[49] and as such, actually more or less contemporary to George. In this chronicle, George, Lord Latimer, is mentioned among a number of other nobles in a variety of events. None of these mentions carry any indication that the chronicler considered him in any way different or unusual, and most definitely, without the slightest indication that he considered him as any lesser. For all that can be learnt from this chronicle, George never suffered from any mental illness at all, and his behaviour was expected to be the same as that of any other nobleman of his standing.

The most important of these mentions of George in the chronicle is his inclusion in a number of lords who attended Queen Margaret in 1460, during the time that Richard, Duke of York laid claim to her husband Henry VI's throne. The notion of George being able to choose a side, go against the brother who was controlling his lands and nobody actually noting it is somewhat unlikely. However, without any background knowledge as to George being considered to suffer from 'idiocy', there would be nothing for a reader of *Gregory's Chronicle* to even hint towards it.[50]

This could be taken as a sign that George's mental illness, even a mental illness that was considered to be so bad that he was considered unable to have custody of his own possessions, was absolutely not stigmatised and that there was no ramification to suffering from such an illness at all. In fact, going by that chronicle alone, it could be concluded that he was treated as if he were entirely healthy despite that, but this is rather far-fetched. Even if absolutely no stigma was attached to suffering from mental illness, it is all but impossible to consider a man both unable to control and manage his own possessions while at the same time able to make far-reaching political decisions. His inclusion in *Gregory's Chronicle* as one of the men serving Queen Margaret nine years after his 'idiocy' had him declared unable to take care of his possessions and basically returned to the legal position of a minor has two possible reasons. One of these is that his mental illness was so low-key that the chronicler was not aware of it, and upon hearing reports as to his presence, he saw no reason to doubt them. However, once George had been officially declared mentally too unwell to take care of his lands, it would have become at least somewhat widely known. Other, similar, cases certainly show that such news did travel fairly fast, even if they did not always excite a lot of interest.

The more likely and rather more pedestrian explanation is that the writer mixed up George with his son, Henry Neville, who was known to have sided with Queen Margaret.[51] This would be a sensible explanation as to why George was mentioned in this chronicle. If so, sadly, it does not further our knowledge about George's life after his brother took over the management of his lands for him.

Though the evidence is very scant, many historians, such as Clark and Burke, have pointed out that what there is suggests that not only George's lands, but also he himself, was taken care of by his family. His first guardian appears to have been his brother, Richard, Earl of Salisbury, and after Richard's death his niece, Alice, Baroness FitzHugh and his nephew Richard, Earl of Warwick took over the position.[52] This would have been a very natural decision to make on everyone's part. There was, however, no official order that made George the ward of any of them, nor were there any restrictions on George being able to go where he wanted and do what he wanted, beyond the obvious pecuniary restrictions of no longer being able to access his own lands and possessions for money. Since Salisbury, and his son Warwick after his death, controlled his lands, it would be only fair if they also housed George and his household, paying for it with his own money, that was in their own hands due to his mental illness.

Both Salisbury and Warwick had very large households, so it is very hard to know if George and his men lived with either of them. It is known, though, that there was never any complaint. George himself might not actually have been in the position to make any complaints, but nor was there ever any complaint from his son either, or any accusations of mismanaging George's lands or keeping them from him when he was once more able to actually manage them himself. Once he was stripped of his lands because his mental illness, of whatever nature it was, became too bad for him to manage them on his own, he never did recover fully, and possibly never actually recovered at all.

Equally, it is possible that he did actually recover to some extent after 1450. Late 1450 is the first time we have evidence for him suffering from some sort of illness, if only by assumption, as he was not invited to parliament in November of that year.[53] While some lesser nobles never were, it was all but unheard of for nobles who had previously been invited to parliament, as George had been, to not receive an invitation, and was only done in some very few cases. There was always a very sound explanation for this, and it stands to reason that the explanation in this case was George starting to suffer from his mental illness.

However, if that was the reason, there is a suggestion he became somewhat better afterwards, for he was invited to parliament again from 1453 onwards,[54] though it is all but impossible to find out which of the lords invited to parliament actually attended it. Technically, it was forbidden to not attend parliament once one had been invited, but not enough evidence survives to find out if this was always adhered to. Notably, however, the exception to this duty to honour the invitation was if the nobleman invited had a sound explanation for his absence, such as an illness.

Usually, such illnesses were physical, but a mental illness would have doubtlessly been accepted just as much. However, as he was not himself his brother's ward and could decide for himself where he went and what he did, the invitation cannot have been purely nominal, and not intended to actually be taken up by George. There would have been absolutely no way to stop George from taking up the invitation, turning up to parliament and wanting to be part of the proceedings. If indeed he was so mentally ill that he could not control himself and was unable to make any sound decisions, such an invitation would not have been issued. Therefore, while still not able to manage his own lands, perhaps due to it being a never-ending task, and a rather stressful one, he was considered sane enough to attend parliament two years after he had been stripped off his lands.

Whether he actually did attend, we do not know, though the suggestion is that he did not.[55] Even so, even if George actively decided against it because of his own mental illness, this suggests a certain self-awareness and as such, indicates that his illness was nowhere near as bad as Henry's, or William Beaumont's. Suggestions could be something like depression, which he would without a doubt be aware of but which would not stop him from usually thinking rationally and even knowing that in his position, it was a bad idea to get involved in politics.

Even so, unless the very fact of George losing his lands is considered punishment, there is no evidence of George in any way suffering any consequences of his mental illness, apart, of course, from the consequences brought on by the mental illness itself. Socially, it does not seem as if it made him an outcast, or that he was thought less of by his family and peers.

1.2. Suicide

In the above-named cases, those affected by mental illness obviously suffered, but none of them, from what we know, tried to kill themselves. There may have been an attempt in the case of William Beaumont, but if so, it was not recorded, quite possibly for a good reason. Suicide was a very different issue from mental illness, and one that was therefore treated differently. It is often assumed that the mere attempt was enough to exclude someone from society, but again there is evidence to show that this was not always the case.

Two typical cases which happened in late mediaeval England are those of William Beaumont's friend, John de Vere, Earl of Oxford, and John Beaufort, Duke of Somerset.

John de Vere's case is less a definite instance of mental illness and more an example of the misconceptions of how mediaeval people dealt with some of the fallout of such illnesses, in this specific case, suicide and suicide attempts.

In many ways, the lives of John de Vere, Earl of Oxford, and his friend William Beaumont were not only similar but overlapped. Four years younger than William, John was considered a more warlike man than him, but even so, it cannot have been easy for him to be involved in battles from a very young age. Being, like William, staunchly Lancastrian, John was initially pardoned by King Edward IV for his involvement on the Lancastrian side. However, by 1468 he had decided on joining some Lancastrian discontents, and spent some time imprisoned for it that year. During the Lancastrian readeption in 1470/1, John was involved in the government, and took part in the Battle of Barnet. Upon being defeated, he fled to exile together with William Beaumont. As mentioned above, the two of them engaged in piracy together in 1473 before they were caught and imprisoned in 1474 and held until they escaped ten years later.

There is no evidence as to how William reacted to this imprisonment, but there is one very telling instance known about John's reaction. In a letter written on 25 August 1478, Sir John Paston told his brother, also called John Paston, of gossip he had heard of crimes committed, of his quarrel with the Duke of Suffolk, and finally of John de Vere's actions at Hammes Castle, which he recorded very drily:

> 'Item, as for the pageant that men say that the Earl of Oxford has played at Hammes, I suppose you have heard thereof; it is so long ago, I was not in this country when the tidings came, therefore I sent you no word thereof.
>
> But for conclusion, as I hear say, he leapt the walls, and went to the dyke [moat], and in to the dyke to the chin, to what intent I cannot tell; some say, to steal away, some think he would have drowned himself, and so it is deemed.'[92]

There is no further information available about this, not even the ruling Sir John Paston alluded to by saying it was 'so [...] deemed'. Again, though, it is interesting that there was no outcry, either at the time or later, when John became very prominent in Henry VII's government.

According to Paston, it was widely known about, but if the tone of his letter is any indication, mostly treated as gossip.

No other mention of the incident has survived, but that, in itself, could be indicative. If suicide was as loathed and regarded as absolutely unforgiveable as is often assumed, then using his supposed suicide attempt against him would have been the obvious course of action for his enemies, or anyone jealous of his position at Henry VII's court. Even if John could explain, or even prove, that he had actually tried to escape, that suicide had never crossed his mind, the very fact he is on record as having attempted suicide, that according to Paston, an official ruling had declared it so, should have been enough to use for anyone trying to attack him. This never happened; in fact, after 1478, there is no evidence his supposed suicide attempt was ever mentioned anywhere again.

Though we cannot say how bad the gossip about it was at the time, and what the feeling about John's supposed suicide attempt was, Sir John Paston is very matter of fact about John's actions, simply detailing them. That he mentions that 'some say' he was trying to flee and 'some say' he was trying to kill himself suggests it was a hot topic that many talked about, but there is no condemnation in the tone in which he records the fact that it was ruled a suicide attempt.

This might not mean very much, as Paston is also very matter of fact about other bits of news he relays in his letter as well, not using any words to indicate any outrage even when reporting a crime a man called William Brandon had committed. However, while there is no open condemnation, the tone the letter uses in this instance is worth comparing to the tone used when discussing John's action:

> 'Item, young William Brandon is in ward, and arrested for that he should have by force ravished and swivved an old gentlewoman, and yet was not therewith eased, but swivved her oldest daughter, and then would have swivved the other sister both; wherefore men say foul of him, and that he would eat the hen and all her chickens, and some say that the King intends to sit upon him, and men say he is like to be hanged, for he has wedded a widow.'[93]

Obviously, William Brandon was considered unforgivable, with men 'say[ing] foul of him' while Sir John does not mention any judgement made on John de Vere by those gossiping about his actions. This is of course very understandable for modern minds, but it is often assumed that suicide was considered worse than anything else. This judgement is understandable: in ecclesiastical law, it was the worst crime. No matter what other crime someone committed, it was considered God's decision whether He could forgive or not, while a suicide was definitely eternally damned. However, the very language Paston uses in his letter about John de Vere and William Brandon, as well as the treatment of William Brandon as compared to John is very telling as to the reality of this. The ecclesiastical law was a theory, while in practice, suicide was not actually considered anywhere near as terrible a crime as things such as rape or murder.

In fact, even the Church does not seem to have been anywhere near as harsh as their actual laws concerning suicide may lead a researcher to think. There is no evidence whatsoever that John had any difficulties with the Church following 1478. It has to be pointed out that from the time we have records of that sort of thing for him, he was a high-ranking noble, but this was not usually a deterrent for churchmen when they condemned someone. There are plenty of examples of churchmen speaking against high-ranking nobles in fifteenth-century England, often calling them sinful, and in some cases, actively condemning them. In fact, there are several examples of nobles who died excommunicate for a variety of reasons, from being a rebel, such as William Beaumont's father John, to being a bad influence, such as Piers Gaveston.[94] These reasons were usually a pretext for hard-nosed political considerations, but they show that there was no hesitation in accusing and even religiously condemning high-ranking noblemen. A reluctance to do so cannot have been why his supposed suicide attempt was never used against John.

Another example for how suicide was treated in late mediaeval England is the case of John Beaufort, Duke of Somerset (1404–1444), a man a generation older than William, Viscount Beaumont and John de Vere, Earl of Oxford. He was the second son of John Beaufort, Earl of Somerset, who was himself a son of the controversial match between Katherine Swynford and John of Gaunt, Duke of Lancaster. John Beaufort the elder had begun life as an illegitimate child of a prince's, but after John and Katherine's marriage, he had been made legitimate by a papal bull.[95]

His parentage means that John Beaufort the younger was closely related to Henry IV, Henry V and Henry VI. Even so, there was nothing particularly unusual about his early life. As he grew older, however, he gained influence at court and was eventually given important military posts. However, he did not show himself to be particularly talented at the tasks he was given. On the contrary, his professional career is one of failures, and evidence suggests it to have been one of these failures that triggered his mental illness.[96]

In 1443, John was given the difficult task of commanding the English troops in their campaign in France. The developments in this war had not been good for the English forces for a while by the time John was given the task, and many historians think that there was no other option but failure for him.[97] After all, the English had been steadily losing all they had won in the previous decades, especially under Henry V's cruel but successful leadership, for at least ten years by that point. Even so, John was to prove singularly inept. Others before him had failed at the task; others after him would, too. None failed quite as spectacularly as he did. This was in part because John chose what could be described as rather pointless tactics with no stated aim,[98] and accepted money to free French prisoners[99] undoing what little successes he had had. However, John's ability, or lack thereof, as a military leader is not the focus of this book. It is simply needed as an explanation as to the circumstances of him becoming ill.

John's failure as Henry VI's battle commander was the last straw for the already strained English forces and Henry VI's already very pro-peace government. Henry VI considered the loss caused by John, or at the very least overseen by John, as leaving them with only one option. Consequently, he chose to listen to some of his most important advisors such as William de la Pole, Earl of Suffolk and decided that it was time to try and make peace with France. The peace was to be made in the time-honoured fashion of monarchs: by arranging a marriage, between King Henry VI and the niece of the King of France, Margaret of Anjou.[100]

Since much of English politics had been focused on this war in France in the years before, and quite a few English lives had been lost in it, this was not a very popular decision. Though in the years to come, it was mostly William, Earl of Suffolk who would be blamed for it; at the time the decision was made, John, Duke of Somerset was also seen as one of the culprits. Though he had not been involved in the decision making, his failure as a commander was seen by some as the deciding factor in Henry VI's choice, and as such, he was shunned. Not only that, but he was actively persecuted for his financial decisions while in France. Moreover, according to the *Croyland Chronicle*, there were 'attempts being made by the servants on his life', and, as a final indignation, he was 'accused of treason' and 'was forbidden to appear in the king's presence'.[101]

It is understandable that such trying circumstances could trigger a mental illness. Even if he were to steer clear of actually being condemned for treason and being executed for it, he must have known that it was the end for any and all political ambitions he had had. John appears to have considered this a terrible fate, at least by the *Croyland Chronicle*, which reported that 'the noble heart of a man of such high rank upon his hearing this most unhappy news, was moved to extreme indignation; and being unable to bear the stain of so great a disgrace, he accelerated his death by putting an end to his existence, it is generally said; preferring thus to cut short his sorrow, rather than pass a life of misery, labouring under so disgraceful a charge.'[102]

Again, the lack of violent condemnation when making this claim is notable: quite obviously, the writer of the chronicle disapproved of what he considered John's choice, but despite this chronicle being written by a clergyman, he does not actually state any of the consequences that John, by ecclesiastical law, faced.

One of those consequences should have been that he was not buried on hallowed ground. That this was not followed in John's case, and he was instead given an honourable burial can presumably be attributed to his family paying a lot of money to the Church so this could happen. Even so, there was no way they could have stopped anyone from speaking about the suicide, and the *Croyland Chronicle* proves they did not. Nor would they have been able to stop any clergyman from condemning him in writing. That the chronicle's author did not must have been a personal choice, his statement about John's suicide perhaps reflecting his own opinion.

Interestingly, it has long since been claimed that John was ill before his death.[103] This theory is somewhat supported by the Croyland Chronicler's statement that John 'accelerated' his death, though this could also simply have meant that he chose to bring it about rather than waiting for the natural end of his life without implying it seemed to be close.

However, that there was a connection between physical and mental health was a belief that was quite widespread in the fifteenth century and might have contributed to the startlingly non-judgemental report of John's alleged suicide in the *Croyland Chronicle*. What this shows is that melancholy — depression in modern terms — was seen as a very real danger to physical health as well.

This connection between mental and physical health is often claimed to have only been found out in the twentieth century, in the later part of the twentieth century at that,[104] but that it was considered a normal, uncontroversial belief can be seen in the announcement made after Henry VI's death. Henry died either on 21 or 23 May 1471, and his death is usually assumed to have been murder on the orders of Edward IV. Since Edward had regained the throne only recently when Henry died (after half a year of Henry being back on the throne), it was assumed, at the time as well as today, that Edward wanted to run no more risks. Henry VI's only son had also recently died, leaving no obvious heir to his dynasty and making the by then elderly Henry the only obvious focal point of rebellion. Consequently, it has often been stated as a matter of course that he did not die of any natural causes but was instead killed. The fact that Henry is known to have suffered a head wound shortly before his death has often been used to support this.

However, even if that is the truth, it is obvious that Edward would not have openly said so. Instead, the explanation given for Henry's death, repeated in *Historie of the Arrivall of Edward IV in England and the Finall Recouerye of his Kingdomes from Henry VI AD M.CCCC. LXXI* was that 'of pure displeasure and melancholy, he died' after 'the certainty of all which [...] came to the knowledge of the said Henry'.[105] By this knowledge, this source meant the fact that Henry's only child and son had died in battle three weeks before, and that his wife had been taken prisoner.

There were many contemporary sources which did not believe this, such as the *Warkworth Chronicle*, which outright stated Henry had been killed.[106] Even so, it is notable that nobody openly rejected the explanation of Henry's melancholy as in itself unbelievable or stupid. It stands to reason that nobody would have said so openly and opened himself up to the possibility of retaliation by Edward IV, who would not have been kind to those accusing him of regicide. Even so, there would have been nothing to stop anyone from pointing out the unlikelihood of such a cause of death had it seemed out of the ordinary to anyone. Moreover, it would hardly have been any more dangerous than outright saying, as chronicles such as the *Warkworth Chronicle* did, that Henry did not die of natural causes.

The obvious conclusion from this is that melancholy was in fact seen as a dangerous illness, an illness that, through affecting the spirit, could also harm the body, causing physical ailments and illnesses, up to and including death. The only reason why it was not accepted for Henry VI's death was that the circumstances of his death were apparent to everyone and did not in fact suggest he died of natural causes at all.

There is another comment about melancholy, and how it was seen in the fifteenth century, in the fact that Edward IV selected this excuse for Henry VI's death, which suggests that one of two scenarios happened: either Henry VI actually did die of natural causes, said by one of the king's physicians to have been caused by melancholy, or else Edward figured it was the most believable lie for Henry, the one that would be least challenged.

It would be a mistake, though, to connect this too much with Henry's mental illness. While it was something that must have been considered, and a death like this would have been stupid to assign to a man known to have been mentally very stable, this does not have to have been the main reason as to why Edward chose it. In the formal explanation of Edward's government, a much more straightforward reason was given for Henry's melancholy, as mentioned above: the recent death of his only child and son.

The end result of this is that it gives a very clear picture of how melancholy was seen in the fifteenth century: it was considered an illness more likely to afflict those already prone to mental instability such as Henry, as it was considered at the time, and it was an illness that could be dangerous. Evidence suggests it was considered likely to be triggered in those prone to it by traumatic events, such as the death of a child or, in the case of John Beaufort, Duke of Somerset, a catastrophic failure or blow of some sort. Once someone suffered from it, it could even kill that person.

Moreover, and perhaps most importantly, in itself, there is little evidence that there was actually stigma attached to it. It was mentioned as a dry fact in sources, without any statements as to any failure on the part of the sufferer. It was treated as something that might hit someone unexpectedly. That this also opens the whole question as to the understanding of mental illness and who, in the fifteenth century, its most likely sufferers were thought to have been, is a question that will be discussed below.

Melancholy is a special case, somewhat different from other mental problems. While other mental illnesses were sometimes treated kindly, as discussed above, they do set apart the sufferers, as the sufferer of a physical illness would also be; melancholy is much more regarded as a fact of life. It is very much treated like something that, under the right circumstances, anyone might get. This, quite possibly, also explains the downright accepting attitude, especially compared with what the laws actually were, both secular and ecclesiastical, of suicide. It was seen as a horrible thing to do, as indeed it is, but the attitude as to why is very similar to our modern attitude, simply with an added religious component. It was not seen as something that a person was ostracised from society for attempting; on the contrary, evidence is clear that help was offered. It was simply seen as something that no one should ever do.

However, all the above examples have been of men of the nobility, men who by birth and marriage had much more influence than most people. By definition, we have less evidence for the lives of commoners, and therefore also less evidence for how mental illnesses were treated in those who were not of the nobility. Even so, there is some general evidence for the treatment of mental illnesses found in physicians' bills, records for what, in modern language, would be called mental hospitals, and chronicles speaking about it. Though there are few, if any, personal stories of any commoner so afflicted known and preserved, certainly there are indications of how it was dealt with and seen in general.

Perhaps not too surprisingly, the gentle treatment that noblemen and noblewomen received was not always visited on commoners with the same or similar inflictions. In their case, the result much more often resulted in being shunned from society, in some cases even being mistreated, and certainly in mockery. Such cases are found, for example, in the records of York and London.[107] The language used in these cases is much more derogatory than seen in the cases of Henry VI and William Beaumont: words such as 'lunatic', 'idiot' and even 'complete idiot' can be found all over the records when dealing with such cases.[108]

As these quotes show, the consequences of suffering from a mental illness were harsh for a commoner, much harsher than for a noble. In some ways, this is understandable, since unlike nobles, most commoners did not have money to fall back onto in case an illness like that made them unable to work. This would result in much straightened circumstances and, as such, may have been a trigger for any mental illness to get worse.

This is not the only difference between commoners suffering from mental illnesses and nobles suffering from the same. Acceptance among their peers was also much lower; and attitudes towards the inmates of Bedlam Hospital could be actively hostile.[109]

Mental illness was not just dangerous in itself; it could also lead to attacks, crimes we would call 'hate crimes' today. This suggests that the acceptance shown in the cases of the high nobility suffering from such illnesses is deceptive and was not shared by the population at large.

It has to be pointed out, though, that there is of course a bias in recording, in favour of nobility and working against commoners. The illnesses of men such as William Beaumont were presumably not well known to the population at large; those who knew of it may very well have voiced derogatory opinions about him and his illness, which were simply not recorded for prosperity. Similarly, while we know of the kind treatment given to nobles suffering from mental illness by their closest circle of friends and relatives, we have no such knowledge in the cases of most commoners, though logic dictates that they were just as kind and understanding as the friends and relatives of ill nobles were, with strangers being far less understanding. The biggest problem for commoners, in this case, would have been that they were not protected from such strangers in anywhere near the same way that noblemen and noblewomen were.

This has to be borne in mind when discussing the subject of suicide. We have seen that nobles who attempted suicide were generally not treated badly at all, and often did not suffer any consequences. Even the memories of those who actually succeeded in killing themselves were not always treated badly, with their family sometimes not suffering any consequences. It was different for many commoners, with the stern consequences we usually associate with suicide in the Middle Ages usually being visited upon them, and superstitions being attached to it not happening.

Again, many such cases are found in the records, and not just in England. In fact, one particularly notable and well-recorded case happened in Basel in June 1439.[110] A woman called Frau [Mrs] Beringer, suddenly taken with a spell of madness, jumped off the roof of her house one night, killing herself. Due to her being a respectable member of society, her parish priest decided to bury her in consecrated ground,[111] but this was a decision that was not popular. When, after her burial, it rained for a week, many citizens considered it was due to Frau Beringer's burial in consecrated ground, and eventually, the case was taken to court.[112] Five days after her death, the body of the unlucky woman was dug up and disposed of by being thrown in the Rhine.[113] When the rain stopped soon afterwards, it was taken as a sign of God's pleasure that a wrong — burying a woman who had killed herself in consecrated ground — had been righted.[114]

Once more, this is not the only such case. Many others are found, some with people expressing similarly strong feelings about the remains of suicide victims, some where they were in fact quietly interred in consecrated ground. In almost all such cases, the feelings of the general population, if recorded, were similar to the feelings known to have influenced the Beringer case. In this instance, the similarity of the shared Christian values overrode any cultural differences between England and Switzerland, or in fact England and France or England and Spain. Moreover, it is notable that almost all recorded suicides by commoners were done in such a way that seemingly nobody witnessed it, even when witnesses could not have stopped the act. Such acts, found in the coroner rolls, are often explicitly stated to have been performed in such a way because of the shame it would cause, and were treated as shameful. One example, found in the coroner's rolls for the year 1322, of a John of Ireland, stated that he was found 'dead of a death other than his rightful death'[115] after he had hanged himself, and that upon discovery of his body, there was concern with his possessions and if they should be confiscated. Therefore, it can be concluded that harsh treatment on the remains of a suicide victim, and even their family, could be considered the norm for commoners, in a startling difference from the nobility.

In many ways, as in this case, it was money that made the difference, with those who could afford to often greasing the palms of the coroners and churchmen. However, there is one problem with this: as historians, we can only work with the evidence we have, and not with something that was hushed up. This sounds self-evident, but still makes a difference. For example, John Beaufort's death was not officially considered a suicide, but natural causes. If he had been a commoner, this is where it would have ended; no chronicler would have been interested in a commoner's death by accident or sudden illness. However, with him being high-born, there was speculation. Therefore, it is quite possible that there were in fact many commoners who did in fact commit suicide, but for whom it was hushed up, as it may have been in the case of John Beaufort and others.

Conversely, there is a case to be made that it would never have happened had John Beaufort been a commoner, and he would have been treated like poor Frau Beringer and John of Ireland in the examples discussed above. However, that is sheerest speculation, and speculation that is not supported by what scant evidence there is. Though there are a number of suicides ruled each year in the coroner rolls[116] there are also some which were ruled strange accidents, with suspicion attached[117] or ones that were simply recorded as accidents but almost certainly were not, as it would have been all but impossible to die accidentally in such ways.

This suggests that it was not just nobility for whom it was attempted to gloss suicides over as much as possible. Perhaps, it would be wrong to say that such attempts were made for commoners 'as much as' for the nobility, as there can be little doubt that money helped hush up possible suicides, but it can be seen that there was always an effort not to rule a death a suicide if it could be at all avoided.

This, in turn, indicates that the cases of John Beaufort, Duke of Somerset and John de Vere, Earl of Oxford, were not exclusive to nobility. Most of the commoners whose death was ruled as suicide might therefore have simply been so obviously a suicide it was hard to hush it up or see it as anything but. Though doubtlessly, it would always have been easier for a member of the nobility to get their relatives' death ruled of natural causes, it does not seem it was entirely a privilege only for them.

Even in the cases of a suicide being said to be such, the language in the coroner's rolls is not as condemning as could possibly be expected. On the contrary, it is very dry, in much the same way as John Paston's statement about the Earl of Oxford's possible suicide attempt and the Duke of Somerset's possible suicide. This is partly because the coroner's rolls are not a chronicle, not supposed to give any value judgements — but only partly. It is very notable that in some cases, a certain judgement is made, even in the case of accidents. Some of these are described as 'foolish', such as the suicide of a man called Henry, who 'by a spontaneous, or rather foolish, death he put an end to his life'.[118]

That no such judgement is made in the case of most suicides does not mean they were accepted. Instead, it was simply widely known that suicide was a mortal sin, but in most cases it was not considered necessary to explicitly stress this, to pour salt in an open wound, so to speak.

On the whole, what can be said is that treatment of commoners and of the nobility, when they suffered from mental illnesses, was both dramatically different and yet equally similar. Commoners would, by necessity, have been more closely associated with people who did not always want the best for them, and would not have been as well protected from those wishing them evil as nobles suffering from mental illness would have been. Moreover, they would not have had the money to fall back on if a mental illness made them unable to function as a worker, and to afford care as seemed necessary. Even so, the attitude towards the causes and the illnesses themselves was, in general, remarkably similar.

Chapter 2

Treatments for mental illnesses

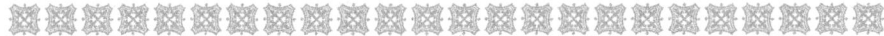

2.1. General treatments

Another aspect of mental illness, though, would not have differed as much for nobles and commoners: the treatments used to cure such illnesses.

The most common association with such treatments during the late Middle Ages is of them being painful and humiliating, an association that is, for modern readers, one that is correct. This is not just the case for cures and treatments recommended for mental illnesses; in general, medicine was nowhere near as advanced as it is today, and therefore often treatments were recommended by physicians that we know today are not just unhelpful but, in many cases, actively harmful such as leeches, blood-letting and head purges.[119]

None of these treatments are a myth; all of them were used against physical illnesses. As such, it is easy to assume that the treatments used against mental illnesses, which are less easy to grasp, would have been even worse. This is not necessarily the case; in many cases, the same sort of treatment was used for both mental illnesses and physical ones.

Due to Henry VI's illness, we actually have a fairly good idea of what treatments were used in England, for a mental illness such as he had. Thankfully, a list of proposed treatments for Henry's illness survives; treatments which appear to have all been administered to the king, and information pertaining to them for the later part of the year 1453 and the year 1454, the years during which the unfortunate king was catatonic.[120]

While treatments ordered by him and administered to him survive for several other years of his reign, it is hard to work out from these just which of these treatments were meant against symptoms of his mental illness, and which were used against physical ailments. It was normal for monarchs and their spouses to be constantly surrounded by physicians and treated for even the most minor illnesses. Therefore, under normal circumstances, it would be hard to work out which recorded treatments were for Henry's mental illness and the symptoms thereof, and which were fairly normal treatments for small physical ailments. Since Henry was catatonic for most of 1453 and all but a few days of 1454, however, all the treatments given to him in that year were, by necessity, at least somewhat connected with his catatonic state.

It is notable that a lot of these suggested treatments are very similar in fact, to treatments used for physical ailments: laxatives, baths, gargles, blood-letting.[121] Others are more obscure, and though similar language was used for physical illnesses, the medicine they actually referred to may have in fact differed somewhat: 'soothing medicines', 'waters', 'syrups'.[122]

This similarity of the treatments suggested to cure Henry's catatonia to treatments for physical illnesses was not due to any lack of differentiation between mental and physical illnesses, but actually well-thought-out logic: the belief was that a diseased mind could not heal in a sick body. The supposed uses for the treatments suggested to Henry have not been recorded, though, so that we can only guess from their usual intended uses what they were meant to achieve. Blood-letting was intended to restore balance to the four humours of the human body, a theory that will be discussed below. Soothing medicines were intended to stop any worry or melancholy which might hinder a recovery. 'Head purges' were intended to relieve the pressure on the head, laxatives thought to remove any harmful foods from the body, purges for a similar reason.

None of these worked, but they do show an interesting understanding in how mental illness worked. Most notably, it was the basis of all these supposed remedies that mental illnesses were caused by ailments of the body. As we shall see below, it was not the only cause of such illnesses that was considered common at the time, but it was the most widespread, and it was the one most cures were based on.

Looking at the treatments given to Henry VI, the explanation favoured for his state was that his body was in some way overworked; too much pressure on his head, too much blood in his veins, too much food in his stomach. That the treatment for a king for a mental illness so severe was based on such very basic premises can be seen as both alarming and as a better understanding of the human psyche than mediaeval physicians are usually credited with.

It is alarming in a way that nobody considered that a mental health condition might need different treatments than a physical health condition. It is equally alarming that, upon them not working, Henry VI's physicians considered that they had not yet found the right treatment rather than coming to the conclusion that none of the rather basic treatments actually worked. Moreover, though this would not have been known at the time, several of these treatments would not have even helped much against a physical illness and might have actively made Henry VI's physical state worse.

On the other hand, the very fact that Henry's physicians connected his mental state with a physical ailment shows that they had an understanding of at least some concepts of mental illness still shared by modern physicians. It is accepted by almost all those who focus on mental illness that mental wellbeing is closely connected with physical wellbeing.[123] Henry's case was an extreme one, in which simply physical cures would be unlikely, even today, to have any success, but the understanding was still there.

Moreover, as horrible as some of the treatments sound, they also show a basic understanding of both physical illnesses as we know them today and the root of mental illnesses. The most obvious example for this is the suggestion of 'head purges', which meant drilling a hole in Henry's head to let some blood out. Though it can sound like ineffective cruelty,[124] it is not too different from some operations performed even today. Though in modern times they are not used to cure mental illnesses, such surgery is still used for the exact same reason Henry's physicians performed them: to stop internal bleeding that could pressure the brain. Such surgeries are obviously done differently today, and exclusively for physical problems,[125] but the concept is very similar.

Though there is no evidence of Henry having any internal bleeding, the idea that too much blood in his head might put pressure on his brain was what was behind the procedure, and it shows that a connection was made between his brain being affected and mental illnesses.

This is, in itself, not indicative of common mental health care in England. Henry VI was king and as such, had access to the best physicians and the most advanced health care available at the time, for physical as well as mental complaints. His treatment does not mean that such was available to all or even most others who suffered from similar mental health issues, or mental health issues at all.

However, even though this is fairly obvious, there is a suggestion that all those who could afford any care at all for their mental illnesses or the illnesses of their neighbours, family and friends, were treated similarly. Though the doctors might not have been anywhere near as skilled as those of King Henry's, the principle of the treatments appeared to stay the same. The records still surviving of mental hospitals such as the Bethlem Hospital (known as Bedlam), in London,[126] show this. Blood-letting, purges and other treatments of the sort were normal, and administered to those who came to be treated, though naturally not all of these treatments were given to all patients.[127] In fact, there was a clear distinction of which treatment was administered to which patient, though since hardly any symptoms are recorded, only the treatment, it is hard to make any guesses as to what was chosen for which illness, or symptoms.

In fact, the case of Bedlam shows several problems with the study of mental illness, and the reception of mental health in the Middle Ages. The first is that it is largely overshadowed by what happened in the centuries afterwards, which was often worse than what happened during mediaeval times. The reception of Bedlam is a very good example for this, as it was an esteemed hospital for mental health in the fifteenth and sixteenth century, with royal patronage and even partly attended by royal doctors.[128] However, the treatments offered became much worse in the centuries that followed,[129] and this has coloured the impression of the hospital as a whole. Stereotypes about the Middle Ages in general have not helped with this impression, with the assumption being that everything became better in the centuries afterwards. This has caused several works on the history of mental health to assume that the horrible circumstances of the seventeenth and eighteenth centuries were actually an improvement to the circumstances during the Middle Ages,[130] though actual primary sources suggest the opposite.

One problem with early research on hospitals is inherent in its nature. The treatments given in Bedlam Hospital caused many people to assume the hospital was thought less to cure mentally ill people and more to punish them for being mentally ill. This assumption has very much coloured the idea of how mentally ill people were viewed in late mediaeval England. Of course, this is viewing everything through a modern lens and is not actually true.

As we have established above, such treatments were even given to King Henry VI, obviously in the hope of curing him, or at least lessening the symptoms of his mental illness to such an extent that he could function well. There is no reason to think that the physicians at Bedlam did not visit these treatments upon their patients with the same aim, not to maim them or punish them, but to try and cure them. That this often did not work was not due to negligence or even an attempt at punishment, but simply because these treatments, though much more considered than we often give physicians of the Middle Ages credit for, were simply not suited as a cure to such illnesses.

The actual effectiveness of the treatments used for mental illnesses and mental health issues will be addressed in the next chapter, but as regards Bedlam Hospital, it is worth mentioning that in the fifteenth century, it was well regarded. In fact, not only do several primary sources attest to it,[131] this can also be seen by the fact that it was led, at times by a royal surgeon. When Edward IV was king, he made his favourite physician, William Hobbes, Master of the hospital.[132] Hobbes was an esteemed physician in addition to a surgeon, and his work at Bedlam Hospital appears to have been considered not only important but groundbreaking.[133]

Moreover, it is a fact that Bedlam Hospital was a flourishing hospital, with many patients. Many of those patients were brought there by their family, and while some of them may have done so to be rid of the responsibility and stigma of being associated with them, the fact that the hospital asked for fairly steep fees[134] makes this unlikely as a general motivation.

The fact that the fees were so high meant, naturally, that very poor people could not hope to afford it and would be left to their own devices to deal with their mental health. This does not take away from it that such a mental health hospital not only existed but was actually under royal protection. It meant that at least for commoners with some money, there was care if they were mentally ill. It also means that not only their friends and relatives cared enough for them to want to see them cured, but also that even the nobility were interested in seeing as many cured as possible.

This, however, does not account for the fact that 'Bedlam' would eventually become a synonym for chaos,[135] and that while the hospital was well regarded, it was still the victim of attacks and hate crimes occasionally. This, too, has been taken as evidence of the widespread rejection of mentally ill people in the Middle Ages and early modern times, but evidence suggests it is only part of the picture. It cannot be denied that mentally ill people faced discrimination at the time, and while sadly this is still sometimes the case today, it was rather more widespread at the time.[136] This will be discussed in Chapter 5. However, as we have seen, it can also not be denied that many people were eager to see mentally ill people treated well and, if possible, cured of their illness and that the efforts to see this was the case for as many people as possible went into the highest echelons of society. Similarly, there were those who mistrusted and mistreated people who suffered from such illnesses, particularly if it made them behave in ways considered strange or unnormal. And there were those whose friends did not think any less of them and did not consider it any worse than a physical illness, something unpleasant that they simply had to deal with.

As has been established above, there were many places to see someone who was suffering from mental illnesses treated. For most people at the time, there were two particularly important pillars of support: physicians, if they could be afforded or otherwise persuaded to treat the patient, and the Church. One very pervasive myth is that the Church, even more so than the general population, rejected those who were mentally ill and sought to only punish them. Again, as much as for the rest of the population, it is only part of the picture. There were religious ramifications of mental illness, and in many cases, those were actively discriminatory.[137] On the other hand, there was equally religious assistance for those so afflicted.[138] In some ways, the attitude of the Church reflected that of the general population: it varied widely. This makes perfect sense if one does not regard the Church as a large monolith, but as an institution consisting of humans, who had a variety of different sets of values and beliefs.

This is easier to understand by realising there was not one set of rules on how to deal with those who were mentally ill. The only set rule was that suicides were excommunicate.[139] As seen above, however, while the rule itself was one that was set in stone, it was one that was, if at all possible, not enforced. In many cases, other mental health issues were also treated in the best possible way for the sufferer, not used as a way of accruing power for the Church.

Looking at the part the Church, or more specifically churchmen, played in the treatment of those who were mentally ill presents the researcher with problems. The first of these is that doing so requires trying to form a complete picture from the bits and snatches that can be found about these issues from primary sources, church books and similar sources. Secondly, one is faced with a variety of stereotypes and later formed prejudices against mediaeval religion, which have to be sorted through to work out what is truth and what is only a myth.

Solving the first problem is difficult in itself already. It is often more difficult than working with secular sources, since not only have many sources been lost but a lot of sources pertaining to the Church have deliberately been destroyed. This happened a lot during the Reformation, as well as afterwards by historians or others with an agenda of trying to make the Middle Ages look as backwards as possible. In many ways, such attempts have been successful, as can be seen by looking at what has been written about mediaeval treatment of mental illness, and especially the supposed attitude of the mediaeval Church towards mental health and mental illness from the eighteenth century onwards. From such writings, it is not hard to gain the impression of mental health issues being actively encouraged to then be used against the hapless mediaeval believer, and to turn the believers against each other, so all the more to rely on the Church.

This idea is widespread and found especially in books written during Victorian times, but to find the truth, one needs to dig deeper. While doubtlessly containing nuggets of truth, the books are not only very general, but they also ignore the other side of the coin, which is that the Church was often a source of support and strength for many people.

To a lesser extent, the same is true for the treatments offered by physicians. As has been seen earlier, it is a very common myth that physicians at best were clueless, using treatments that had no chance of succeeding on patients suffering from mental illnesses. At worst, the physicians are presented as having been actively malignant, trying to punish these patients, oftentimes with the active support of their friends and relatives.

Any work on mental health and mental illness in the late Middle Ages must therefore be concerned with sorting through such prejudices and finding out how true they are. This has to happen in addition to looking at what treatments were offered and how helpful or not they were. It is also important to attempt to humanise not only those suffering from mental illness during the Middle Ages, but also their surroundings: their clergymen, their physicians, their friends, relatives and neighbours.

Most significantly for this study, as there is the most evidence about it, there was also a whole host of secular treatments, offered by actual physicians who also dealt with more prosaic physical illnesses, for mental health problems. In fact, these treatments often overlapped, due to a belief that many mental illnesses, if not caused by any religious problems, were in fact caused by physical ailments.

This is a startling belief, which is in some ways still echoed in modern medicine, in which self-care is stressed, and constant physical illness is recognised as a very strong trigger for mental illness.

Naturally, modern medicine has progressed with the treatment of such mental illnesses, as it has progressed with the treatment of physical illnesses. However, that connection between physical and mental led, in the late Middle Ages, to the idea that most mental illnesses could be cured, if at all, by medicines that also helped physical illnesses.

While this sounds as if these treatments relied mostly on guesswork as to what mental illness could be connected with what physical ailment and therefore what treatment should be chosen, it was somewhat more refined than that. In fact, medical books of the time did discuss the treatment of mental health issues as a separate issue. It was not always considered to have been started by a physical ailment, as will be discussed.

In some ways, the fact that mostly treatments for physical ailments were chosen was a sign of helplessness, a sign that nothing else was known that could be helpful for such mental health problems. The idea of talking therapy it is not a modern one, but as established above, this was much more a treatment offered by the Church, with priests often working as what today would be called psychologists. If, however, a mental health issue was taken to a physician, there would be a physical treatment offered.

These were not always as brutal or as shocking as the treatments given to Henry VI suggest. Henry's case was an extreme one, and as such would have been considered to require extreme actions, for two obvious reasons. The first reason was that his symptoms were not just occasional in 1453, but rather constant, with recovery being the only aim and the only chance to return Henry VI not only to coherency but to functionality. Second was the fact that he was king. While certainly, seeing to it that a friend or loved one was cured would have been of just as much importance to any commoner as it would have been to Henry VI's loved ones to see him cured, a king being so ill had ramifications for the entire kingdom. As such, the most extreme treatments would have been used.

For everyone else, and even for kings and nobles less strongly afflicted, there were other treatments, treatments which even to a modern mind promise more success. These had a lot to do with the famous idea of the body being made of four humours, and that an imbalance of these humours could cause not only physical illness but also an imbalance of spirit. These four humours were blood, phlegm, black bile and yellow bile,[140] and each of these humours, or fluids, was connected with a personality type: sanguine, phlegmatic, melancholy and choleric. While it was accepted that every person was different, with some leaning more towards melancholy and others to a phlegmatic nature, it was considered that if there was an imbalance caused by something, these traits would become more extreme.[141] If they became too extreme, they would make a person mentally ill. A melancholy person might, for instance, despair of life itself; a choleric person might, like Henry VI's grandfather, Charles VI, become murderous.[142]

To prevent this, there were some fairly easy measures in place, some of which sound barbaric to us while others sound like common sense. An example of the former is what was done in the case of someone who was considered too sanguine, which was meant to indicate too much blood in comparison to the other humours.[143] The solution was the most famous of mediaeval treatments, for physical and mental illnesses alike: bleeding a patient, and as such removing the supposedly surplus blood from the body.[144]

With our medical knowledge today, it is hardly surprising that this did not work. However, it was seen as a success that often, due to the loss of blood, the patient fainted. Since this was seen as a sign of the body reacting, it was seen as proof that it worked, at least in the short term.[145]

A similar, and similarly gruesome, treatment was used for a supposed excess of yellow bile, by the theory of the four humours leading to choleric behaviour. The most logical solution to that was removing the supposedly surplus yellow bile, much like the supposedly surplus blood was removed in the case of too strongly sanguine behaviour. The patient would receive an emetic, so he or she would vomit, as such removing all the bile.[146]

Again, it is not particularly surprising that such a treatment did not have much long-term success. However, the treatment for a surplus of black bile, considered to lead to melancholy behaviour, was much more mellow and much more in sync with what today would be recommended for depression, if not as a sole treatment: a change in diet.[147]

In fact, interestingly, what was recommended as healthy for a person suffering from excessive melancholy — in more modern terms, a person suffering from depression — was what even today would be seen as a very healthy diet: a diet with a lot of vegetables, especially salad, which was seen to absorb black bile.[148]

This did not cure any depression, but the healthy effect of a good and balanced diet even on mental health issues has long since been proven.[149] It is therefore not surprising that similarly good effects were noted by mediaeval physicians treating patients for melancholy.

This system is often presented as very clear-cut, with patients falling into any one of those four categories and classed as being too melancholy, too choleric, too sanguine or too phlegmatic. In reality, there were cases in which such a distinction could not be so clearly made. This appears to have been the case with most men and women suffering from mental illness. Only very rarely could they be sorted explicitly into only one of these very narrow categories, and the mentally ill usually were not put solely into one of them.[150] Some mental illnesses could cause a person to be in two, on the face of it, rather contradictory categories. Someone suffering from what we today would call bipolar disorder would, for example, be both choleric and melancholy, with either of the treatments designed to calm one side being considered to bring out the other side more. Sadly, there is very little recorded for such cases, though there are suggestions that in the event of something like this happening, the illness was considered more severe, and therefore more severe treatments were used.[151]

One such treatment was, again, bleeding,[152] which was not only used to remove 'surplus' blood, but also to treat physical illnesses such as fever. Laxatives, emetics and similar were equally used, with varying success.[153] In some cases, it was advised to do nothing at all. This would have only been possible if the patient were either restrained or in an environment where he or she couldn't harm anyone, either themselves or anyone else.[154]

Such spaces were rare. For commoners, it would have been nearly impossible to find a place where they could be alone like this. Unlike what we today are used to with private spaces in our own private flats, there would have been no such space for mediaeval commoners. Even for nobles, this would have been all but unheard of. Even the most high-born noble was always surrounded by servants and would have been expected to show himself or herself, to live their lives more or less in the spotlight.

Therefore, the only place where such a private space could be provided was a mental hospital, such as Bedlam. As mentioned above, in the late Middle Ages this was an institution with a very good reputation, considered to be very helpful to those suffering from mental illness. However, as also mentioned above, there was still a lot of prejudice against the hospital and its patients. Part of this was based on the notion of 'madmen' or 'madwomen', as they would have been called then, being given the run of the place and not actually being treated correctly.[155] In short, the stereotype, on which such prejudices were based, was that there was no real treatment being undertaken, because such 'real' treatment would come with real restrictions, often presumably physically bad ones.

This is in itself telling about the widespread assumption of how mental illnesses should be treated. Conversely, it also shows that in some mental hospitals there were no such restrictions and the mental health patients were not actually restrained in any way. Only those who were dangerous were. Evidence for that survives. In such a case, if someone was criminally insane for instance, or feared to become so, the treatments in Bedlam were harsh,[156] as they were in any other mental health hospital at the time[157] and for a very long time afterwards.[158] In the records we have of Bedlam Hospital, there are mentions of patients being chained to the walls, so they would not be able to harm others.

Patients in the grip of delusions who were harmless, however, would not be so restrained. Since it was considered the most promising treatment to just leave them alone until the delusions had passed, this was the policy followed in Bedlam Hospital.[159] Again, this sounds less than helpful to modern readers, with our modern knowledge of medicine today, but it can hardly be denied that in the face of the alternatives, of invasive physical treatments which would hardly have helped, this was the best course of action.

The prospect of a cure was pretty dire even following this course of action and many of those who could afford it stayed in Bedlam Hospital for the rest of their lives once they had been brought there or voluntarily admitted themselves with mental health issues.[160] Only very few were ever considered cured and released. However, it should be said that even today, many mental health professionals believe that a cure of mental illnesses is all but impossible.[161] The current theory is that at best, they can be controlled both through medicine, which would not yet have existed in the Middle Ages, and therapy, which did in its most basic form.

Such understanding did not exist in the Middle Ages. Failing to cure such issues was usually regarded as a failure on the part of the physicians by contemporaries, who did not share our understanding of the difficulty, if not the downright impossibility, of curing mental illnesses for good. The expectation in the fifteenth century, for example, was that if a physician treated someone who suffered from delusions or was catatonic, he would cure him for good, as he might cure someone of a physical illness.

This was an expectation not only held by laypeople, but that was shared by many, if not all physicians. It is known, for example, that Henry VI's physicians worked with the aim of completely restoring their royal patient's mental health, so that he would never suffer from any mental illness again. In fact, when Henry woke from his catatonic state on Christmas Day 1454, there was not only a hope but an expectation he had fully recovered and there would be no relapses.[162]

Under such expectations, any treatment could not help but fail, even if it were the most brilliant treatment, which most of the treatments offered by mediaeval physicians were not. However, neither were the treatments, both secular and religious, all completely terrible and useless. Some were in fact helpful, at least in the short term, and some achieved results, even if not in the way such results would be expected today.

It would be interesting to see if the rates of success were better for physicians working for the prevention of mental health issues. This is something for which it is very hard to find any data for, as it was a very obscure discipline in the late Middle Ages. There are almost no details on any specific cases, which is unsatisfactory and leaves any researcher to simply look at the theory and make some speculations.

While this means there can be no statement made about the effectivity of such measures of prevention as were suggested during the late Middle Ages for mental illnesses, we can compare the advice given in medical books to advice we follow today. This enables us to make a very interesting comparison as to how these issues were seen today as compared to several hundred years ago.

As is to be expected, such care was mostly concerned with keeping the humours in balance[163] and were as such mostly recommendations for physical wellbeing. Most of these pieces of advice were very close to the treatments administered to people who were suffering from symptoms of a mental illness that was considered to be caused by an imbalance of these humours, as detailed above. Especially with those who were considered to be prone to a melancholy mood, there seemed barely any difference in how prevention and actual treatment of an already existing condition worked. A healthy diet was still recommended, including many vegetables,[164] something that we can imagine worked at least somewhat well. At the very least, it is still part of mental health care today. Even in cases where it does not work, what can be said is that nobody has yet invented a better way of preventing such illnesses as depression.

For cholerics, prevention was not the same as cure, as it was not considered a sensible measure to stop an excess of yellow bile by vomiting pre-emptively. In fact, in this case diet also played a part; a diet that stressed other parts of what today we would call the food pyramid: meat. The logic was that in the same way salad was supposed to soak up the excess black bile, meat was meant to replenish any lack of blood, and hence restore the balance between the excessive yellow bile and the other humours.[165]

Unsurprisingly, it was the same for the other two humours, phlegm and blood, as well, with certain foods meant to counteract the excesses. This was only a rudimentary idea of health care, but just how successful it was, we have no way of knowing. Apart from the use of salad to heal depression, which echoes several of our own medical ideas, it really sounds more like quack than medicine. Even so, at the very least the idea of food being very important to mental health and a good diet possibly preventing mental health issues is an interesting one. It is purest speculation how this was received, though, and if it did help with mental health and prevention of mental illness at large. It could be argued that there was a good chance of such prevention measures succeeding at least partly, as much as mental health issues can be prevented with what would today be termed 'self-care'. After all, there is a good chance that most people, as discussed above, would not simply have felt they were strictly part of one category, but would have considered normal changing moods as evidence they had an excess of one humour, then an excess of another. This could have very well made them not binge on one recommended food but vary between any of the recommendations, with the result being a balanced diet. This, at the very least, would have worked for prevention of the physical illnesses now often associated with the Middle Ages, and as we know from modern-day studies, might also have helped against depression, if nothing else.

There was, however, also a flipside to this: the possibility of someone believing they actually did fall squarely into one of those categories and only following the recommendation for this explicit category. This would result in terrible overeating of only one food group, which would lead to physical illness and as such, if not actually cause mental health problems, at the least not actually prevent any. The fact that such a mistake would have almost exclusively been made by someone who was already prone to suffering from some sort of mental illness, for example those suffering from melancholy, would have made this worse. On the face of it this could have led to some harmless, if not helpful, advice becoming actively malignant. However, in the absence of contemporary statements about these ideas, all we can do is judge it in the same way that modern day suggestions and measures would be judged.

In some ways, it appears that this was also how these measures of prevention were judged at the time: simply by seeing if, and how, they worked, and, if necessary, adjusting them accordingly. This was done several times that we know of, so that the treatments offered for several mental health issues and mental illnesses changed over time.

This change of treatment during the Middle Ages is a fascinating subject in itself. Most of this book is concerned with the late mediaeval period, during which the treatments were already rather advanced when compared to the preceding centuries. The early and high Middle Ages were not quite as advanced, and it was from that time that many of our misconceptions come from (if not from the Georgian and Victorian periods). In the eleventh century it was considered hardly unusual to lock away those who were afflicted with some sort of mental illness, so as not to 'embarrass' the family.[166] This discriminatory behaviour was not simply confined to mental illnesses, nor was it confined to the high Middle Ages, or really the Middle Ages at all, but it is notable that we have far more evidence for that sort of behaviour for that time than we do for similar behaviour in later centuries.[167]

Perhaps not surprisingly, the actual treatments given by physicians at that time were also harsher and generally more painful than they were later on. Procedures such as patients being tied up, physically hurt and, especially in the case of female patients, being sexually assaulted,[168] are recorded as having taken place far more often. Again, this is not solely confined to mediaeval times, and in fact, there is a case to be made that it became worse in later centuries. In fact, in the nineteenth century, what can only be classed as sexual assault was used as a treatment for women with certain conditions, while in the Middle Ages, it was seen as a crime, if sadly one that was not considered particularly terrible.

For all this, mental health hospitals already existed in earlier centuries and were, for example, well established during the fourteenth century in England. This seems somewhat contradictory, in that there was a concern for mentally ill people despite them often being seen as simply an embarrassment, a liability not to be mentioned. Even so, the mere existence of these hospitals challenges these preconceptions, and suggests that mentally ill people were in fact regarded as an ill friend or family member in as much need of treatment as those suffering from physical ailments, and that while societal perception was harsher than in later centuries, personal perceptions were not.

Mediaeval mental health hospitals are often claimed to be proof of exactly that supposed harsh and judgemental view of the mentally ill; of people wanting to 'be rid of' their 'embarrassing' mentally unwell or ill relatives and friends. It is clear by looking at the broader development of acceptance of mental illnesses that the opposite is the case. So, as discussed above, is the way these mental health hospitals were structured. They were not meant to punish or lock the patients away from the world, but on the contrary, they were meant to cure the patients, even if the very fact that this was rarely achieved clouds the picture somewhat.

Just by looking at the treatments used against all sorts of mental illnesses, we can tell that by comparison to what had been done in the centuries before, during the early and high Middle Ages, the cures suggested and used during the fourteenth and fifteenth centuries were fairly enlightened. While during the eleventh and twelfth centuries, there appears to have been a lot of what today we would call 'shock therapy',[169] this was no longer the case in the fourteenth and fifteenth centuries.[170] The treatments are perhaps shocking to us but at the time were perfectly normal ones that were also used for physical treatments, and some explicitly used for mental health issues, which, as stated above, at least shares the general ideas with treatments mentioned above.

There is a certain reflection of the progress of society found in the research of how mentally ill patients were treated in society as well as explicitly receiving treatment in a medical context. During the eleventh and twelfth centuries, much was based on earlier texts, by famous physicians.[171] This was not to change much in the later century, but something happened in the twelfth century that has since been termed the Renaissance of the High Middle Ages by scholars: a renewed interest in Roman and Greek texts.[172] While these had never completely gone out of fashion, there was a very limited pool of those texts available to physicians especially during the early Middle Ages. With the advent of more universities, this changed. Roman and Greek texts were not so much rediscovered as became fashionable again,[173] and more ideas from them were taken up. Mental illness has been a phenomenon since the dawn of time, so there is also a lot to be found on it in medical texts from the Roman and Greek era. As more of these texts became widespread and read by those who could all over Europe, more ideas were included in the general use of physicians. It was around then that mental health care became a much more widely accepted phenomenon.[174] Nor were the conclusions and ideas from these old texts blindly accepted. There was a lot of experimentation done, there was debate about it, and as always in such scientific subjects, this caused progress, and so it did for mental health care.

There was another benefit of more universities existing all over Europe, a benefit that especially concerned medical sciences, if not solely so: it encouraged more travelling and therefore more mixing of cultures, bringing together different ideas. It has long since been known that during the Middle Ages there was a lot of progress in particular in medical sciences in the Middle East. Though the supposed squalor of Europe has been exaggerated to the point of ridicule,[175] while the supposed enlightenment of the Middle East has equally been somewhat exaggerated,[176] there is no denying that European physicians benefitted significantly from the exchange of ideas with Middle Easterners coming to see European universities, studying and teaching there.[177]

That there was any one particular idea with regards to mental health and the treatment of mental illnesses that was accepted explicitly from a Middle Eastern source is hard, if not impossible to say, but it certainly stands to reason, given the influence of Middle Eastern ideas on medicine as a whole.[178] We do know that in these centuries, mental health care and the treatment of mental illnesses made an enormous leap forward,[179] and while there is no concrete evidence of the correlation of the influx of Middle Eastern ideas being the cause of this, it is a fairly logical conclusion.

What can be said from this is that changes in society as a whole also reflected on the treatment of mental illnesses, in more than one way. The acceptance of mental health increased much more, though it was far from a utopia (even today it still isn't) and the actual medical treatment improved much.

2.2. Religious treatments

Medical treatments are obviously all physical in some way. However, during the Middle Ages there was another very important section of treatment: religious ones.

In our secular age, any religious advice for healing any sickness, physical or mental, is at best scorned at, at worst used as evidence of the Church's malignant nature. However, this was not seen the same way in the Middle Ages, and it would be a mistake to dismiss the healing power of prayer, if only as a way of calming people down.

In fact, it is recorded that in some cases of mental illness, for example what we today would call paranoia and depression, prayers offered help to those afflicted by them. This is not particularly surprising, as it could have given the sufferers the feeling that they were not alone, that someone — God, in this case — was on their side, and that all their struggles could be eased by Him if He so chose. Even today, while prayer is rarely offered as a treatment in itself, it is considered very important in cases of paranoia, depression and similar illnesses to shift the focus onto good things, and for the sufferer to remember that there are people on their side.[180] In some ways, offering prayers was much the same, especially if done together with a priest. Such help would, by mediaeval understanding, have meant that they were twice as likely to be heard by God.

Because religion and the Church were a constant in almost everyone's life in mediaeval England, as well as France, Spain and the rest of Europe, it would probably have been where most people first turned when they had problems. Physicians were costly, even if they worked in hospitals that charged little and made allowances for those not rich enough to afford good care. The only hospitals in which poor people could even hope to be treated, if they were unable to afford the fees charged by others, would have been run by monasteries and convents, and were, as such, also connected with the Church.

This would have been something that the majority of people at the time were aware of, and everyone would have had access to their own priest, even if this priest may very well have only been a village priest, not a far better educated bishop or other prelate. By necessity, even such simple priests had to have a certain education. Due to this, in many places priests were not only considered the theological experts, but they also acted as helpers with many other issues. This, of course, gave them immense power, and many of them misused this power, but it was not always the case. In many cases, they readily used their influence to help others. A great case for this is St Francis of Assisi, who was actually explicitly started to work with those insane.[181]

Since all illness, physical and mental alike, was considered in a certain way to be a punishment or a test from God[182] — a concept that will be explored in more depth in Chapter 4 — a priest would have been the obvious person to contact if someone was struggling with their mental health. This appears to have been a concept that was widespread all over Europe and is found in sources written in England as much as in sources from France, Spain, or other parts of Europe. Thus, reacting to a mental health issue by turning to a priest would presumably have been a reaction that was the same everywhere. It is definitely known that contacting a priest with such problems was a common and accepted occurrence in England in the late Middle Ages. Nor would it have been difficult for anyone to find a priest. In general, a village priest was a fixture in many people's life, there for baptisms, weddings, last rites, funerals, and often sent for when someone was ailing. In many ways, having trouble with mental health would have only been another illness for a priest to address.

This is backed up by evidence, although there are very few specific cases of commoners struggling with mental illness recorded before such illnesses escalated. However, though there is a sad lack of personal detail, we have more wealth of information where treatments the Church might have offered is concerned.

A stable, perhaps the most common piece of advice was, of course, prayer. Again, like most of the treatments addressed earlier in this chapter, this was not something that was only advised in the case of mental illness, but was generally recommended, whatever someone was ailing from, whether it was a physical or mental illness.

Another treatment often offered to those afflicted by mental illness was the suggestion of a pilgrimage.[183] This would, however, have only been a treatment available to those who could afford to leave their hometown, as well as those whose mental illness did not totally incapacitate them, the way Henry VI was incapacitated. However, again, for those suffering from depression, it was often considered a good treatment.

Again, though it sounds rather strange to modern ears, it was a treatment that was actually fairly successful. In important places of pilgrimage — Our Lady of Walsingham and Thomas Becket's shrine in Canterbury in England, for example, as well as Santiago de Compostela in Spain, and naturally Jerusalem — many prayers for help are recorded, as well as prayers of gratitude. These are often concerned with illnesses, and often with mental illnesses as well. A good example for this is Santiago de Compostela in Spain, with many miracles helping the mentally ill recorded there, and it was a popular destination for English pilgrims.

However, in some ways, religion could also be dangerous for those suffering from mental illness. Some of the treatments suggested by priests were actively dangerous, even if they were not actually intended to be so, much less to be a punishment of any sort. It was a staple of mediaeval religion to react to any problem, be it of a secular or a spiritual nature, by offering something to God, to show the strength of devotion. This could be something like fasting or spending all night at prayer,[184] something that would be uncomfortable for healthy men and women but a risk for those already ailing. This particular spiritual solution highlights a big difference between those afflicted by physical illness and those suffering from a mental illness. It was known, even at the time, that such devotions could be actively dangerous for those suffering from physical illnesses.[185] For this reason, not only were physically ill people actively discouraged from performing them, in many cases they were excused even from rituals usually demanded from everyone, such as not eating meat during Lent.[186] The exceptions recorded in the Papal Calendars were only available for rich men and women, who could afford to pay for such indults, but while less recorded, there is evidence that even village priests could judge such situations and gave permission for pregnant women and other people in peril of becoming sick or more sick to abstain from these religious occasions.[187]

However, there were no such indults and no such permissions for those suffering from mental illnesses, despite the fact that at least some physicians were aware of the connection between physical and mental health. Not only that, but there is evidence, found in the Papal Calendars among other sources, that more fasting, more devotions and other physically exhausting exercises were often recommended as treatment for mental illnesses.[188] In many cases, this not only did not help, but actively made the illness worse. A typical example for this would be someone suffering from delusions or hallucinations, which is a condition that can be made worse by hunger, exhaustion and other physical problems actively caused by fasting and long devotions. That this happened occasionally we know from several miracle stories connected with the sites of pilgrimage mentioned above.[189]

Another issue surrounding mental illness and religion was recognising what actually constituted a mental illness. This was not a problem that was solely concerned with religion, and in fact, many secular lords and commoners had similar problems. While some mental illnesses were easily recognisable as such, such as Henry VI's illness or that of his grandfather, the French king, Charles VI, who reportedly believed he was being followed when in the throes of a spell of his illness, others were not as easily recognisable to mediaeval men and women.

Hallucinations and auditory hallucinations were such cases. To modern readers, it is obvious as a very clear symptom of a mental illness, though which one cannot always be diagnosed and understood by a layman. During the Middle Ages, it was equally obvious as a religious experience of a sort. This very conviction has, in fact, been used as a centrepiece of condemnation against the mediaeval Church; evidence of clergymen using mentally ill people to further their own aims. It has sometimes even led to commenters to speculate that 'the Church' deliberately caused hallucinations. This, however, presupposes that these clergymen had complete modern understanding of these mental health issues, while nobody else did, an assumption that is absurd. Since it was not known at the time what caused mentally ill patients to hear voices — it is, even today, something that cannot be entirely explained and is hotly debated among mental health experts — mediaeval men and women, clergymen included, simply explained these issues in the only way they could: by considering it to be caused by either God or the Devil, depending on the situation.[190]

There were precedents to people at the time believing it as many religious stories mentioned such experiences, and featured saints hearing the voices of other saints, or of angels.[191] Nor was it a belief only shared by commoners, somehow manipulated by clergymen. There is every bit of evidence that not only did clergymen, even those of high standing such as bishops and cardinals, and even popes actually believe it, but that so did kings, nobles and, perhaps most importantly, physicians more concerned with more secular treatments than prayers and pilgrimages also shared the same belief.[192]

The most famous case of someone hearing voices in the Middle Ages is Joan of Arc, the commoner girl who rose to fame and power in the early fifteenth century, who was eventually burned at the stake for heresy. Her case is an excellent example of the exploitation of mental illness at the time, how differently it could be received, as well as the understanding of God and the Devil shared in the Middle Ages, and how it was connected with mental health, mental illness and the treatment thereof.

The story of Joan of Arc is explored in depth in biographies of her, attempting to reconstruct her life from the many myths and legends surrounding her. The most recent of these biographies in English has been by Helen Castor.[193] However, by necessity, neither that book nor any of the others written about her have a focus on whatever Joan's mental health issues were. While the fact that she heard voices is mentioned, and some speculation as to what illness might have caused these symptoms is included, the focus lies on her actions.[194] However, especially for any analysis of her death, it is important to remember that to have a justification for her execution, Joan's mental illness was used against her.

In fairness, it would not have been considered like this by any of the men who condemned her. The very fact that she was said to hear voices commanding her to do what they said, while a clear indicator of madness for any modern reader, was not considered such by the English forces any more than it had been by the French.

It was considered either divine or satanic interference, or else, an attempt to fake such an interference.[195] It was this that the English forces accused Joan of, but as it happened, they did not succeed in making Joan show up any inconsistency in her story.[196] In the end, poor Joan was executed for heresy, not for claiming to hear saintly voices, as was doubtlessly what had been originally planned, but simply for wearing men's clothing.

Joan died at the stake on 31 May 1431, condemned to death by the English forces against whom she had fought, and not saved by the French king for whom she had fought. Her case became widely known through this, but perhaps more interesting than the military aspect is how very differently French and English forces treated Joan's claim of hearing saints' voices. This, of course, makes Joan's case particularly fascinating for a study of mental illness: Joan's actions directly influenced the politics of both England and France and were therefore discussed in both countries, making her a very rare case in which the same case was analysed at the same time in two different countries. This showcases not only the obvious political opinion about her, but also the cultural stance towards cases such as hers.

In the light of this, it is particularly notable that no sources in either France or England stated that Joan was a 'madwoman', as would have been said at the time. They both took this statement of her as matter of fact, with the French sources, understandably, treating the voices she heard as evidence of divine support, or her being directly led by God and his saints.[197] The English sources, however, saw it differently, with one version being that she simply pretended to be hearing these voices,[198] claiming to have knowledge of saintly advice she did not in reality have. Another view, that first became popular in the decades after her death and was carried over into later centuries, was that she had in fact been a witch and that the voices she had heard had in fact been conjured by her, and as such were devilish, rather than divine.[199]

The language used in English sources is naturally rather hostile, while French sources are much kinder about her. Neither of the two countries, however, saw Joan as mentally ill. This proves that while in many ways there was a more widespread knowledge of mental illness than we today give the mediaeval world credit for, in other ways there was a shocking lack of knowledge in many areas. Many illnesses we know today are mental health issues were not necessarily seen as such at the time.

The very fact that one of the most common symptoms of mental illness, hearing voices and hallucinations, were not actually considered symptoms of mental problems but rather as a whole separate issue, as a religious experience, meant that people suffering from them would not actually be treated in any way. In some ways, it was thought to be a natural occurrence and if the voices were 'only' telling the sufferer what to do, it was in fact sometimes considered a sign of particular piety.[200] It was a different case if the voices were violent, which not only made the sufferer struggle with them, but was also considered a sign that the devil, or demons, had accessed someone's mind, and therefore often seen as a lack of piety.[201] The treatments for this were often, once more, signs of piety, of debasement towards God. These signs could be fairly simple donations towards a shrine or simply to the Church,[202] which was in some cases doubtlessly an exploitation by the Church, but would not harm those who could afford it any further. Other treatments were less harmless, as they would range from fasting to active bodily harm, such as wearing a hairshirt or even whipping themselves.[203] In most cases, these signs of debasement did nothing to cure any mental illness, and if anything, actually only made the voices worse. The end effect was sometimes that people ended up killing themselves with their penance.[204]

On the whole, it can be seen that the influence of the Church and the treatments often offered for mental health problems was not wholly malignant. In some cases, it could offer valuable support which actually helped people deal with mental illnesses. Conversely, in the worst case, it could actively make them worse. In effect, it was just as bad or good at offering treatment for such issues as other, secular, attempts were.

2.3. Suspected causes and how they affected treatments

Measures of prevention only work if there is an idea to work with about what actually causes the illnesses that one wants to prevent. As has been established in the chapters above, despite the reputation of mediaeval medicine, there were actually quite a variety of suggestions as to what caused mental illnesses.

The most interesting, and for modern ears perhaps the most baffling idea was that different mental illnesses were caused by different triggers.[205] It sounds fairly obvious to anyone familiar with twenty-first-century medicine, but the very fact that it was also already known in the fifteenth century shows that mental illness was somewhat better understood than is commonly believed, and that mental illnesses were considered important enough to actually try and find out more about them.

As has been stated above, the most common cause for many mental illnesses and mental health issues was considered some physical ailment.[206] This also explains the whole idea of the four humours, an imbalance of which could make someone both physically and mentally ill, with one in fact often being considered to follow the other. This explained the idea of someone being treated in a gentle way by being recommended to eat better food as well as in a less than gentle way by being forced or fed an emetic, to forcefully get rid of the excess of the offending humour.

As has been seen in earlier in this chapter, which is closely connected with causes, there were even harsher physical measures taken to heal what was considered 'a diseased mind' or 'a diseased spirit'.[207] The reason for wanting to drill a hole in the head — a procedure that sounds much more terrifying than it actually was[208] — was that it was considered that one of the causes of mental illness was that there was too much blood in the brain. This is a diagnosis that is not too dissimilar from the modern one of pressure on the brain, which needs to be prevented by surgery. Though today's complex surgery cannot be compared with the surgery undertaken during the Middle Ages, the idea that such operations instantly led to death is a wrong one.[209] In fact, looking at the surviving records of Bedlam Hospital reveals that there were several such operations done, and the outcome was not always fatal.[210]

However, nor does the outcome seem to have been what was expected. The explanation offered for that appears to have been that the operation had not gone right or had not fulfilled what it was meant to do, not that the underlying cause for the operation was a wrong one.[211] This leaves us with two conclusions. One, that there was not really much flexibility on the idea of causes for certain mental health issues, and two, that the idea of brain damage causing a personality change and certain mental illnesses was one that was already known about during mediaeval times.

It was not that the ideas were completely static, but it is true that such perceptions changed only very slowly, with new information being included gradually. This holds true for both the treatments, as discussed above, as well as for what was considered to cause such illnesses.

As with the treatments, the search for causes of mental illness was much influenced by the renewed interest in old medical texts from the time of the Romans and the Greeks, who had their own ideas which were incorporated into the beliefs of several European countries at the time.[212] This caused something of a shift away from mental health issues being seen as mainly a cause for religious intervention to more of a secular problem.[213] However, as will be discussed below, there was never a complete separation during the Middle Ages and for long afterwards as well. Even so, the inclusion caused more reasons to be considered, and was one of the main reasons for mental health being considered to be connected to physical health.

The influx of people from other cultures in England and France also changed the way mental illness was thought about and what could be considered causes, as they always marked a change in treatment. This is only natural, as with more viewpoints and more cultural ideas around, it made discussion and scholarship around the subject much more varied and inevitably more successful. As discussed above, it has long since been well known that much was learned in Europe, especially under the influence of the Middle East regarding physical treatments, and there was also an interest in Middle Eastern ideas of how illnesses came to be.

Some causes, however, were purely based on observation, without any outside influence. A very good example for this is the fact that it was known, even at the time, that long imprisonment, especially solitary confinement, caused a delay in mental development. This was seen at the end of the Middle Ages and the dawn of early modern Europe, in one very famous example from England: the case of Edward Plantagenet, Earl of Warwick.

Son of a prince, George, Duke of Clarence and nephew to two kings, Edward IV and Richard III, the little boy had been imprisoned in the Tower of London upon the usurpation of the English throne by Henry VII. Due to his claim to the throne, which was doubtlessly stronger than that of the newly made Tudor king, he was considered a danger and never allowed to leave his prison for fourteen years. After that time, he was tried for treason and executed, in what even at the time had been called out as judicial murder.[214] It has been recorded that the boy, who was 10 years old when he was imprisoned and 24 when he was murdered, was all but held in solitary confinement, with nobody but servants seeing him.[215]

At his trial, Edward reacted rather slowly and according to at least one contemporary, who had no reason to lie or be ill-disposed to Henry VII and therefore make up stories to make him look bad, he did not understand what was happening to him, and was in mind still like a child.[216]

In the centuries since, with propaganda to boost Henry VII's name being often taken at face value, it has often been said that little Edward was born 'slow', and was mentally ill,[217] like Henry VI. However, not only does the evidence of his early life not bear this out, but it was also not what was said by the contemporaries watching his trial and execution. These men explicitly stated that it had been his long imprisonment that had left him emotionally stunted, at the level of the child he had been when he had first been imprisoned.[218]

A similar case was recorded around a century later, with another boy of royal descent, although not as close royally as little Edward, Earl of Warwick. This case was another Edward — Edward Courteney. Though only the descendant in the third generation of the sister of a queen, he too had been imprisoned in the Tower of London for a very long time due to his royal blood. When he was finally released under Elizabeth I, he was stated to be 'foolish',[219] to not understand court and politics,[220] and to act more or less like a child or a young teen.[221] Whether it was that or if it was actually being a malcontent, he was drawn into a rebellion, and was eventually executed for it. Though, unlike the innocent little Earl of Warwick, he was definitely guilty, similar comments were made at his execution, of him not understanding what was happening and of him also not having understood the ramifications of the rebellion in which he had participated.[222]

Therefore, it was well known at least during the late Middle Ages and the early modern time that long solitary imprisonment could damage mental health, delay development and have similarly adverse effects, which were irreversible. The fact that this was treated very matter of factly by commenters shows it was not a new or shocking idea, but simply regarded as a fact of life. It is not a difficult deduction to make, but it shows that at the time, simple observations were also taken as evidence for causes of mental illnesses. If the observation were clear enough, and could be replicated enough, as sadly it could in the case of imprisonment, it was taken as a mere fact of life, rather than a theory.

Tying in with this somewhat, the effect of childhood abuse, trauma and other horrible events was also seen as a cause for mental illness. In fact, the concept of a childhood psyche not only existing but being very important for the development of a human being comes from the late Middle Ages. At the very least, it was known at the time, though sadly, it was a knowledge that was lost in later years, in particular in the Georgian and Victorian eras,[223] and was rediscovered only in the later twentieth century.

However, there are not only statements to that effect found in books on medicine dating from the late mediaeval period which show that it was something that was known, but even in famous works often used and referenced at the time.[224] There is also evidence that it was widely known and accepted, rather than simply being a fact known to medical professionals but not accepted by the population at large.

To properly examine this, though, there needs to be an excursion into the understanding of childhood, another subject that is more fraught than it looks. It is a rather strange, if curiously widespread, idea that during the mediaeval period, childhood was not considered its own stage of life,[225] and that due to high child mortality, parents did not love their children to spare themselves the heartache of many of their offspring dying.[226]

If such were the case, there would not be a lot of interest in development and the ways to ensure that no trauma could stunt the emotional development of a child, but evidence does not bear it out. Even though child mortality was catastrophically high, it has been pointed out by many historians in recent years that not only is there plenty of evidence of parents loving their children, but it would also be very much against human nature to assume that parents could simply turn off parental affection. The idea very much rests in a sort of superiority complex often held towards mediaeval people.

More interesting, if one looks at development and how it was viewed with regards to mental health, mental and emotional development and mental illness, is the idea that children were considered small adults.[227] In some ways, of course, as compared to our modern era, they were. There was no choice but for children to face some of the rough realities of life; death, war, famine. This was however not due to a lack of understanding of childhood, but simply the realities of life, which stayed the same for the centuries after the mediaeval period as well. Only in the last hundred or so years have the circumstances of life changed enough, and even then only in some very few parts of the world, for this to be different. At the time, such harsh subjects we try now to shelter children from if at all possible were a part of life that could not be looked away from, for children or adults alike.

Despite this, and the fact that this caused children to grow up faster than is usual in the modern Western world, the idea of childhood not being considered a separate part of life and children being considered as small adults cannot be supported.[228] Nicholas Orme goes into this in detail in his book *Medieval Children*, thoroughly debunking the idea by pointing out that much of the evidence being used for such a claim is otherwise explicable.[229] The book gives a very good overview of what mediaeval childhood would have looked like, and that there was, according to mediaeval understanding, not only a very definite understanding of childhood, but there were also different phases of childhood, which are actually not too different from modern developmental stages.[230]

Orme's book is worth reading for anyone interested in the realities of childhood in the Middle Ages. For a book on mental health, it is simply worth knowing and understanding what childhood meant in the Middle Ages, which was not too different from the understanding of childhood today, allowing for drastically different circumstances of life. As such, it would make sense if contemporary works on mental health made a distinction between the mental health of children and adults, but such distinctions are rarely found. In fact, the only subject addressing mental health that is explored in any medical books of the time is actually how trauma and abuse during childhood can shape a person into adulthood and be a trigger for mental illness.[231] If there was any research done into the actual effect on the actual children, it was either not recorded or such records have not survived.

Even so, the subject on how adults could be influenced by trauma in childhood is one that was actually mentioned in medical texts,[232] although it seemed to treat trauma in children much the same as trauma as adults in how it influenced the psyche. For example, the effect of a child watching someone commit a murder up close was not treated much differently to that of an adult watching it up close.[233] There was only one significant difference: for something that was considered harsh and terrible enough for an adult to not only cause trauma but to be a trigger for mental illness, it was considered that children were more vulnerable to it.[234]

Although in theory it was hard for adults to experience something considered bad enough to cause mental illness, this does not actually have to be the case in practice. It is something that is another myth and, moreover, one that is based on many modern perceptions of something being horrible enough to cause trauma as opposed to something being simply a fact of life.[235] Since, as established above and a fact that is widely accepted, life during mediaeval times was clearly much rougher and harsher than today, the suggestion is that there would have to be extreme trauma for it to be considered bad enough to be different to everyday life.

In a way, this is true. If something is common, it is not going to be a terrible event that makes a change to life in general. But the idea of something that was generally accepted causing trauma was typically not a mediaeval concept. It would be expected that there had to be a general level of acceptance of terrible but normal traumas of life, an acceptance that life was tough in general, and that death and destruction were but a part of it. Given the infant and child mortality, the way that illnesses could kill healthy men and women in the prime of their life without warning, the frequent wars, the fact that food was not guaranteed and famines happened with alarming frequency in Europe during the mediaeval period and to modern minds the unfair feudal system, such an acceptance was simply needed to lead a happy or at least satisfied life.

Even so, this does not mean that those who struggled with accepting some aspects of this were ignored, and even that there was an ignorance of the consequences such terrible features of life could occasionally lead to. In some ways, this is not too different from today. Though life in the Western world has become infinitely better in the latter half of the twentieth and twenty-first century, there are still people to whom horrible life events happen, or those who cannot deal with even the 'normal' vicissitudes of life. This is generally viewed, even today, with some sort of pity and compassion, though it is still not something that is accepted by everyone.

Evidence suggests it was the same way in the Middle Ages. While it was clear that a sort of fatalism was required to live a happy life, and that a thick skin was required to deal with the blows that inevitably happened during life, there was no immediate rejection for those who could not deal with it and who were traumatised by blows most others could deal with. There is something of a suggestion that if someone became mentally ill due to having suffered many blows, there was more widespread societal acceptance, even a degree of understanding, than for most other mental illnesses and mental health problems, for which the cause was not quite so obvious.

Chapter 3

Societal reaction

The best example for this is William Beaumont, Viscount Beaumont, whose case has been discussed in Chapter 1. In his case, it seems it was accepted that whatever his mental illness actually was and whatever symptoms he had in detail, it was caused by the civil war that had been fought on and off in England for the last thirty years before William's symptoms either first started or were first recorded. This is particularly interesting in that William was hardly the only one badly affected by these conflicts, and in fact, many of those close to him had suffered through similar consequences of it. While William had spent nearly twenty years in exile, had lost most of his family during that time without being able to say goodbye and, upon returning from exile, found that one of his nephews, doubtlessly the only family member he could still remember from his time before his exile, was set on fighting against everything William had fought for, this was hardly a very unusual case. Though it sounds harsh to modern ears, it was, and still remains, a feature of civil war to tear families apart and at times even have family members fighting against each other. In fact, William's close friend, John de Vere, Earl of Oxford, had a rather similar experience. He had spent almost the same amount of time in exile as William, having shared prison and other nasty experiences with him, and having lost family members without being able to say goodbye. As discussed above, there is a very clear indication he was badly affected by this too, to the extent of possibly attempting suicide after several years in prison. However, this would have been considered a permanent solution to what John may have figured was a rather permanent problem, and for all the horror of it, fairly rational. William, obviously, did not have that rationality and was very badly affected by what had happened.

In fact, the difference between William and John and their mental health reaction to the very similar situations they had found themselves faced with appears to be that John seemed to have trouble with being powerless, not being able to do anything against the dire straits he found himself in. Once he was himself, as much back in control as he could ever hope to be, there seemed to have been no more difficulties for him to deal with the realities of his life. It seemed to attack his mental health far more to be powerless than dealing with what life threw at him in the best way he could. William, on the other hand, seemed overwhelmed by what had happened during the civil war and by problems that were out of his control, that he could not change, no matter how much political power he had.

This also could have been the reason why, contemporarily, John de Vere was considered mentally healthy, despite his possible suicide attempt, whereas William Beaumont was considered 'mad'.[236] The distinction is very easy for us — William appeared to act rather irrationally, though we do not know exactly in what way, while John seemed to have been perfectly rational and showed no sign whatsoever of suicidal thoughts after having regained power. However, despite the fact that, as we have seen, suicide was often pitied and all that could be done was done to see to it that there was a loophole found to give those who had committed suicide a chance to get into heaven after all, or, failing this, at least shelter the victim's family from the consequences, it was still a mortal sin. An attempt could still be forgiven according to mediaeval theology but was still a sign that the person who had attempted it was mentally unwell, even diseased, even if they had since recovered.

The fact that this was not the case for John de Vere suggests that it was considered, while unforgivable had he succeeded, still a fairly understandable reaction to the situation he had found himself in — a prisoner away from his home country and his family, unlikely to ever be freed. This meant, by contemporary understanding, he had committed a terrible sin, but did not showcase mental illness. William, on the other hand, was obviously mentally ill.

Even so, as discussed above, there was a lot of understanding for that. Not just for his illness as such, and the way his contemporaries saw him, but also for what was considered the cause: a terrible time during the civil war, which had effectively robbed him of his family, of his freedom for years at a time and, it seemed to be considered at the time, his sanity. The fact that at least one source stressed the fact that William Beaumont had been unusually tolerant towards other opinions, stating that he was happy 'let[ting] each man place his feet in the soil as the good lord intended'[237] for himself and what he believed, shows that there was an understanding that unlike many others, he had simply not been made to be a warrior and that he was not the sort of person who could deal with constant warfare and strife.

The fact that this was not only accepted but that his unusually pacifistic outlook was used and accepted[238] as explanation for his mental illness is certainly remarkable and tells us a lot about the understanding late mediaeval English society had of mental illness, and even of its causes.

The most important conclusion is certainly that causes for mental illness and mental health problems were not seen as static, which can be well illustrated in William's case. As a whole, the series of conflicts over who was to have the throne of England was considered regrettable but necessary to defend whoever the chronicler supported against the other, nefarious side. This also meant that in general, everyone who in any way could — healthy men who were not monks or clergymen — should have to fight and do his duty for the rightful king, whoever he thought the rightful king was.

However, while it was seen as that and not as so traumatic that men's minds would give way under it, this was obviously simply a general theory that could be amended to special cases, such as William's. Being considered a very tolerant and peaceful man in contemporary sources, and from what little we know, his actual contemporaries, such as his best friend and his wife, seemed to accept that it had been too much for him in particular.

It could be argued that William's was an exceptional case, possibly because he was an important nobleman or because he happened to be surrounded by unusually tolerant people. However, recorded comments about other people known to be suffering from mental illnesses speak against that theory. The best example for that is the unfortunate Henry VI, whose mental illness and the treatments as well as the reception of the illness in itself have been discussed in Chapters 1 and 2. Comments about his illness and their reflection of the ideas of what caused his illness are illuminating. One of these ideas was that he was simply a very gentle and soft man,[239] not suited to the harsh and often cruel business of kingship.[240] This echoes the theory about the case of William's madness. Both men were considered to be too gentle and tolerant to be involved in extended warfare and deal with the inevitable nasty fallout of it. In some ways, they were pitied for it, though there is no suggestion that it was in any way a reflection on people's general ideas on kingship or war. These concepts were considered important, with Henry and William simply two men not cut out for it and going mad under the pressure that other men could seemingly easily deal with.

There were also other ideas about what caused Henry VI's mental illness as well, both of which are worth addressing as they give an insight into the ideas discussed in the fifteenth century as potential triggers for mental illness. One is an idea that modern medicine has actually proved has merit: inheritance. Since Henry VI's maternal grandfather, Charles VI, himself suffered from a mental illness, there was a lot of language against the French in English sources, of Charles having given Henry his mental illness.[241]

Though a lot of these claims were loaded with anti-French prejudice, and as such this could be read as polemic rather than a genuine attempt to explore the causes of the unfortunate king's illness. They are still illuminating however, as Henry VI never met his French grandfather and could therefore not have been said to have been corrupted by him in other ways. Charles VI corrupting his grandson would therefore have to have been through inheritance, thus showing that the idea of mental illnesses being genetic was one that, if obviously not in these terms, was already one that at the very least seemed feasible in the fifteenth century.

This is supported by the fact that French sources, more hostile towards the English and unwilling to blame their own king for the English king's incapacity unless this was something the French chroniclers genuinely believed in, echoed this idea.[242] That Charles VI had passed on his mental illness to his English grandson was something that seemed widely accepted, and the logic of this was not questioned.

Since we today know that the tendency for mental illnesses is indeed often genetic, this is a fairly astute assessment by the mediaeval French and English. It is also an assessment that could have been based on observation. Though perhaps the most high-profile case, Charles and

Henry were hardly the only closely related people during the Middle Ages who both suffered from mental illnesses. Especially as when they lived, the understanding of mental illness had come on leaps and bounds from what it had been only one and a half centuries before, and there were physicians specialising in it so in some ways, mere observation and records of these observations could have been the cause for this idea.

As such, it is hardly surprising that a certain knowledge of the possibility of inheriting mental illness existed in late mediaeval England and France. It is, however, yet another indicator that the study of mental illness was one that was taken seriously at the time. It also shows that mental health problems were considered actual illnesses rather than simply ignored or that sufferers were ostracised as morally inferior.

However, in the case of Charles VI and Henry VI, there is some doubt as to whether it was really an illness that grandfather passed on to grandson. As Lauren Johnson points out in her biography of Henry VI, their symptoms were very different.[243] She suggests Henry might have been suffering from extreme depression,[244] while Charles's symptoms suggest more extreme schizophrenia.[245] Though other mental illnesses have been suggested for Henry,[246] it is notable that there are no mental illnesses known which combine the very contradictory symptoms these two men showed, or which sometimes manifest in one way and sometimes in the other. Therefore, while there might have been a certain inclination to mental illness being passed on between grandfather and grandson, they do not actually seem to have suffered from the same symptoms.

This has not, however, stopped most historians in the last 600 years from taking this idea of Henry VI's mental illness being inherited from his grandfather as fact,[247] right up into the twenty-first century.[248] Though the theory has been developed further in the last few years, with it being pointed out that even if Henry had inherited the inclination, it would have been triggered by something,[249] the idea in general has stayed the same. This is irrelevant as to the idea of causes of mental illness in the Middle Ages in all ways except one: it shows that in some ways, the perception of mental illness or at the very least the causes of it, has not changed significantly since mediaeval times.

It has to be pointed out that modern-day historians have an advantage over mediaeval chroniclers, in that they have access to documents and physicians' bills and similar evidence about the two kings' illnesses.[250]

This enables them to get a much more complete picture of what these two men were suffering from, though of course, it is still not easy to piece together. The information mediaeval chroniclers would have had access to would have been far less illuminating and often incorrect. It would have mostly been the few snippets actually revealed to the population, and gossip. Therefore, it would make sense for mediaeval English and French chroniclers to think that grandfather and grandson suffered from mostly the same illness. This is particularly the case since they did not live in the same country and at the same time. Though there was a steady flow of information between the two countries, it would have been difficult to get to know exact information even if they had lived at the same time and there was no gossip to muddy the waters. As it was, though, it is fairly obvious why both French and English commenters believed Henry VI and Charles VI suffered from the same illness. Thus, the idea it had been passed on from the latter to the former must have seemed the most obvious and logical one.

Perhaps, it was even one that physicians shared, though that is hard if not impossible to know. However, as to the causes of Charles's illness, it appears to have been considered not to have been caused by any outward circumstances,[251] such as William Beaumont's was; even Henry VI's illness was sometimes considered to have been something of a birth defect. Perhaps due to this belief, there was very little by way of speculation as to the whys and wherefores in French sources, in contrast to the English sources when Henry VI became ill. As to why Charles's illness was seen that way, even though it first manifested while he was already an adult, in very trying circumstances, nothing is to be found.

Another suggestion made contemporarily, as well as in later times, as to the cause of Henry VI's mental illness is a very interesting one, as it goes back to the understanding of childhood and childhood psyche: the suggestion that Henry's mental illness was caused not by inheritance, or perhaps not primarily by inheritance, but by the fact that he became king at the age of only eight months and could not deal with the pressure of this large responsibility when growing up, eventually cracking when it became too much.[252]

This is the best and most clear indicator we have for mediaeval mental health care taking into account the experiences of patients when growing up and factoring these experiences into the causes of a mental illness.

It also shows that there was an understanding that what was suited for adults was not necessarily suited for children and that what was suited for some men and women was not suited for others. This gives an idea of individuality that is rather a foreign concept to most people when thinking about the Middle Ages. In fact, it even stands in contrast to a lot of contemporary mediaeval understanding about society and people. Even so, it does not seem to have been a controversial concept.

That Henry VI was generally not suited to be king and the fact he did become king at a very young age might have been harmful to his psyche is an idea that would square quite well even with our modern knowledge of mental health and mental illnesses. It is interesting, though, that it was a concept that was considered contemporarily in Henry's case.[253] He was hardly the only king who inherited the title and the responsibilities as a child, though he was in fact the youngest English king there had ever been, and, so far, ever would be. Even so, Richard II had become king at age 10, and though it did not end well for him, this was not because of any mental illnesses he suffered from, but because of a variety of other social and political reasons. Since Henry VI was born and became king easily within living memory of Richard II inheriting the throne, this might have been scary for some for these political reasons. The fact that he was obviously too young to rule for several years and, by necessity, protectors would have to do it, was well understood but the precedent case of Richard II gave absolutely no reason to suspect that these circumstances would be bad for Henry VI's mental health.

In fact, this shows that the idea of Henry VI not being able to deal with the pressure of kingship from childhood on, an idea advanced later in the unfortunate king's life, was not just a theoretical one: it was instead based on observation. Observation of children in general and a knowledge of how most children react in times of stress and how they react to too much pressure, but also observation of Henry in particular. It was, therefore, an idea that factored these considerations in but also paid attention to Henry's personality, and as such, shows there was one aspect of mediaeval mental health care that is usually never addressed: individuality.

This is a subject that is important, especially to the religious aspect of mental health, mental illness and how they were received in the Middle Ages. Even so, the childhood psyche aspect of this particular theory for the cause of Henry VI's illness should not be rejected, as despite Henry's personality obviously playing a large part in it, it does not seem like it was considered the most important part of this theory. This indeed seems to have been his extreme youth.

In a way, this is probably best explained by looking at the theory of childhood and its phases in late mediaeval and early modern English society. As has been alluded to, childhood was not just seen as an unspecified time of life before some hit puberty or rather, became an adult, but instead was split into very definite parts.[254] These parts were babyhood, early childhood, age of reason and finally puberty.[255] The age of reason was commonly thought to start at the age of about 7 years old,[256] which was usually also the age children left the nursery.[257] This meant, for high-born children certainly, that they would no longer be taken care of by nannies (called nurses at the time) but would be subsequently taught by tutors. Usually, children also received their first holy communion at around this time, which showed that they were considered old enough to understand the significance of this ritual, despite not yet having the same level of understanding on both religious as well as secular matters as adults.

Richard II had been 10 years old when he became king in 1377, and therefore of the age of reason. Henry VI, however, had been far off that, he had been only an infant and not even able to talk yet. That this made a difference appears to have been widely considered as perfectly clear. Though not yet old enough to rule, Richard II would have understood what it meant, at least in a rudimentary way, to become a king. Henry VI would not, and therefore, he would have always been king for as long as he could remember and would have spent his infancy, babyhood and toddler years aware that he was king, an importance too difficult for a child, let alone a toddler, to grasp.

Even according to our modern understanding, this could have affected Henry VI badly, and evidence suggests that his contemporaries shared this understanding. This means they could also follow that this might be bad for his psyche and could even trigger mental illnesses. The very fact that children were only intended to experience stressful but much more normal ceremonies (such as funerals for a relative) after the age of 7 would have helped this understanding as well.

It appears to have been this understanding that was the reason for Henry VI's coronation not happening until he was 8 years old and therefore had reached the age of reason.[258] At this age, he was considered if not old enough to rule, to at least understand both the significance of his kingship and of the ceremony of the coronation. That he had spent the first eight years of his life already being king, growing up never knowing anything else, seems to have been considered by many of his contemporaries a reason as to why his mind gave way.[259]

The last cause given contemporarily for Henry's mental illness was, in modern terms, inability to deal with failure: in this particular case, not failure of anything he had done himself, but failure at being a king who either won wars or managed to negotiate a successful peace. Henry had, of course, inherited a particularly bad and fraught situation from his father Henry V: he was to be king of France as well as king of England, and defend himself against the French troops supporting his uncle, the French Dauphin.[260]

This situation had happened because Henry V and his troops had been successful conquerors, who had eventually forced Charles VI, Henry's equally mentally ill grandfather, into signing a treaty massively favouring the English and disadvantaging the French. This treaty not only arranged the marriage between Henry V and Charles's daughter Catherine, who became Henry VI's mother, but also stipulated that Henry V would become king of France once Charles died, rather than Charles's son.

Henry V and Charles VI died within weeks of each other, leaving little Henry VI not only with the English kingship but a claim to the throne of France. Naturally, he was too young to even understand this, but since the French heir to the throne was unlikely to take his own disinheritance lying down, and in the event did not, Henry VI's regents saw to it that they continued fighting in his name in France. In 1431, only a little more than a year after his coronation as king of England in November 1429, Henry was also crowned king of France. However, the English war efforts soon started failing, and as Henry VI became of an age to rule for himself in 1437, he was more interested in peace than in continuing the fight. He did appoint leaders for the war in France in his first years as independent ruler (rather than under the guidance of his protectors) but he was not to prove successful at it. Many historians have doubted if anyone could have been,[261] but Henry's contemporaries, not surprisingly, did not see it the same way, many blaming him for always choosing the wrong people to lead,[262] not seeming to show any of the interest his own father had in the conflict in France and even of not sitting on the French throne at all.

As history proved, Henry had no interest at all in this, and finally, in his mid-twenties, decided to end the conflict with a marriage. This was hardly an unusual move to end wars in the fifteenth century (or before or afterwards) but it was not a popular decision in England at the time. Kings making unpopular decisions was hardly unheard of, but Henry was eventually considered to have failed as much at making peace as he had at keeping up a steady war effort with successes for the English. His marriage to Margaret of Anjou, a niece of the French king, brought the English massive losses and only a short-term ceasefire. When the English efforts in France were ended in the 1450s, England was in a far worse position that when they had started after the infant Henry VI had become king.

Again, historians have been far kinder about this than Henry's contemporaries, who saw it as a massive failure on his part that could have been avoided. If this is true is unknown, but for this book, that is not important. What is important is what his contemporaries thought. They did consider it a failure, a failure which caused Henry's mental illness.[263] The logic behind this appears to have been, if we go by the words of Harding's chronicle,[264] that he had caused trouble not only for himself but also for his countrymen by not ruling by himself but instead by being led by advisors. By doing this he had supposedly invalidated the sacrifice of the men who had fallen in France while fighting for him.

To sum it up, the idea was that it was guilt which made his mind give way. This is very interesting in itself, and more so as the very fact he was so high profile caused many people to comment on his mental health issues and propose their theories as to what the illness was, where it came from, and how it could be treated and healed. It therefore gives a fairly good picture as to the ideas and theories of mental health and mental illness as a whole that circulated not only in fifteenth-century England but also in fifteenth-century France.

This last point, of Henry VI being driven 'mad' by guilt, was a widespread explanation for madness, and, as will be seen below, was regarded as a possible cause for madness, usually coupled with religious fervour.[265] As is natural, cases of so-called 'madness' coupled with the suspected cause of guilt can often be found in records of criminal trials. In the fourteenth and fifteenth centuries, there are several cases recorded of men going crazy with guilt after having killed a loved one, such as a wife or brother. Examples of this are found in the coroner's rolls.[266]

This did not engender any sympathy by contemporaries, which is in some way understandable, if still somewhat harsh for modern ears. The madness coming after the guilt was something that was often seen as part of the punishment,[267] and as such was treated with the same contempt as the usually inevitable execution of the offender. However, it was also something that seemed to inspire interest and even made people explore it in fiction, as will be discussed below, in Chapter 5.

There are, of course, also cases in which the 'madness' and the guilt are flipped, for instance someone who suffered from ill mental health accidentally hurting or killing someone while in the throes of this mental illness.[268]

This was not treated the same as someone going mad after committing a crime. There was somewhat limited sympathy for someone who killed or otherwise harmed someone while in the throes of an attack of so-called madness,[269] but there was none for those who went mad with guilt.

The difference can be seen from the documents of trials. As mentioned above, there were several cases in which it was said that someone had gone crazy with the weight of guilt after committing a crime.[270] These men, and in rare cases women, were almost all executed,[271] with no sympathy being given to their state; it being considered a simple consequence of what they had done and as such, their own fault. However, men, and again in rarer cases women, who had killed someone because they were already mentally ill were usually spared execution. In fact, up until 1541, there existed a law in England that said that no insane person was to be executed for high treason.[272]

The very fact that some who had gone mad after their crime were still executed once more points towards the fact that this was not seen as illness,[273] but as mere consequence of the crime. It also pre-empted any plea of insanity to explain a deed.

However, if someone was already known to have been insane at the time they were being charged with something, this law worked for them. This gives us another insight of how mental illness was thought of and how it was treated. Rather than treating those suffering from mental illness and considered 'mad' at the time worse and making them convenient scapegoats for anything and everything that went wrong, the law was actually more lax for them. The fact that people who were not mentally healthy did not understand what they were doing in the same way as mentally healthy people could was considered during trials.

In a way, then, even the law extended some kindness towards those suffering from mental illness, even at a point when this had made them harm others. However, while doubtlessly that was the intention, it was a rather cruel mercy in many cases. Then as now, an insanity plea being believed did not mean that the person so judged was free to leave. Usually, as it does now, it meant being brought to a mental hospital. As established above, these were not the hellholes as they are often described, but those criminally insane were often subjected to very harsh treatment, nonetheless. Sometimes they were chained to a wall, so as not to attack someone, or put in solitary confinement, which resulted only in making these patients' mental state worse.

In some ways, therefore, guilt as a cause of insanity and insanity as a case of guilt show both the best and the worst of mediaeval understanding of mental health, ranging from complete callousness (an understanding that someone who cracked under the weight of guilt deserved it) to a sympathy even extending to the law (although those so afflicted often not being treated with kindness).

This is but a taster of mediaeval understanding of mental health issues and mental illness, and the treatment of many of those afflicted. This has already been touched upon in Chapter 2, but there is another aspect of this: mentally ill people were not expected to participate in society like others. This was, in some ways, a kindness but could also be used against those so afflicted.

This sort of kindness, however, counted mostly for commoners, gentry or the lower nobility. In the case of royalty, an accusation of insanity could do much more harm, as has been seen in the cases of Henry VI and Charles VI, and especially the so-called Juana La Loca, daughter of Isabella of Castile and Ferdinand of Aragon, whose supposed mental illness caused even her family to mistreat her. However, due to the nature of royalty, it was hard to accuse someone of insanity if they were not actually in some way struggling with mental health issues.[274] Though royalty was shielded in many ways from the population, personal appearances were an important part of their duties and it was hard to convince a fellow royal or even the population in general of a royal's insanity if they were frequently seen and always appeared normal.

However, if there was some sort of oddity, a strangeness about how they behaved, or if they were not seen for a while, then such rumours could thrive. Naturally, even kings and queens could and did get sick, and therefore unable to meet ambassadors and dignitaries and be seen by the population for a while. Such occasions, however, were almost always marked by prayers being said for the affected monarch or consort, sometimes with bulletins being issued about their state of health. This was the case, for example, when Edward IV of England caught the measles in late 1463.[275] Though he had only recently come to the throne, usurping the throne from the genuinely mentally ill Henry, nobody seemed to consider that there was anything strange about him having a normal physical illness,[276] and the bulletins as to his illness and his recovery were believed.[277] Though there were still many supporters of Henry VI at large, and would soon prove they were ready to try and dethrone Edward, there is no evidence of any plan to use this illness against the king, to accuse him of being just as mentally ill as Henry, and therefore just as unsuited to sitting on the throne.

This, too, proves that there needed to be more than a momentary and very explicable absence from official duties and from appearances to even start a rumour about mental illness. Even Henry VI's own case shows this very well. When he suddenly became catatonic in August 1453, there was no immediate outcry, no suspicion that anything particularly bad had happened. The first information given to the population appears to have simply spoken of the king being ill, which was accepted at first,[278] like Edward IV's short illness in late 1463 was accepted.

It was only later that rumours about Henry VI's condition became known and then it was through rumour and leaks as well. Unsurprisingly, the nobility learnt very quickly of Henry VI's ill health, though details were suppressed. The nature of Henry's illness could not be kept hidden for long. This was only natural, of course. While in cases such as Edward IV's, he only allowed a limited group of people to see him; there would have been concrete information about what he suffered from even if the monarch in question kept away from people more than was usual. This happened, for example, for Henry VII when he became ill after his wife died in February 1503, when he famously allowed no one but his mother and servants to see him. His court received information as to his status of health,[279] and he still issued orders via his servants.[280]

Henry VI's lack of doing this in August 1453, combined with there being no concrete information as to what was ailing him, quickly alarmed his nobles and made them think that something more than a physical illness was going on.[281] Rumours of mental illness started circulating among them quickly. This is understandable under the circumstances, and another factor in addition to the ones mentioned above cannot be overlooked: the way the nobility worked meant that they were not only interconnected but many had a very effective spy system. Presumably, while there was no official confirmation for a while, the speculation and rumours were stoked by at least one important noble having spies in Henry VI's household who passed on information about his state.

However, there was no confirmation, even for the nobility, until one of the highest-ranking nobles forced the issue: Henry VI's distant cousin and heir presumptive, Richard, Duke of York. Hearing of Henry being incapacitated in some way, Richard had come to court to find he was not being received by the ill king any more than anyone else, and that the pregnant queen and her closest supporters were trying to reign in the king's name. According to legend, Richard insisted to hear the king's confirmation that this was what he wanted to happen during his illness, but he was not allowed to speak to the king.[282]

By this point, everyone must have known that this was not a state that could continue, and that Henry was not suffering from a 'normal' physical and contagious illness. When Richard threw his weight around, he was eventually allowed to see his cousin, who was catatonic, and did not recognise him, nor actually understand what was happening around him, or able to react to anything.[283] In some ways, he was in a coma.

This meant that he could not rule and that someone else had to do it for him, acting as a protector (as had happened during his childhood) until such a time that he recovered.

The very fact that Henry VI's illness was kept a secret for so long has sometimes been taken as evidence that mental illness was seen as shameful,[284] and that it would be bad for Henry VI himself if it was known he was catatonic. There is even a suggestion that this might prevent him from ruling again when and if he recovered.[285] There is a fraction of truth in this. His mental illness was used politically against him even after he had recovered. However, as mentioned above, it was not actually used as a personal attack. Fears of such attacks very probably existed, but they were not the main reason why the nature of Henry's illness was kept secret, even from his nobles, for as long as possible while there was hope of him soon recovering. The main reason was a far more pedestrian one: it was a political disaster.[286]

This is natural and was not due to his mental illness in itself. The main point was that, with Henry being catatonic and unresponsive, England was, in effect, back to the same situation they had been in when Henry had been an infant: someone else having to rule for a king who could give no guidance and could not be relied on as a mainstay.[287]

It was for that reason, the same reason that having a child king was considered very dangerous, that Henry's mental illness was, and has been in the centuries since, considered a political disaster, not primarily due to the stigma on mental illness.[288] As the historian Matthew Lewis put it, the greatest problem was that while Henry was, in effect, back to being an infant king, there was no certainty that given enough time, the situation would be over.[289-290]

Henry being mentally ill, rather than being laid up with a physical illness that took him out of the political game for a while, had another disadvantage: even should he recover, there could always be relapses. Though during the late mediaeval period treatment for mental illness was always geared to complete recovery, it was well known that relapses could and often did happen.[291] While the assumption once Henry had recovered was, as mentioned above, that he was cured, a fear of relapse was mentioned repeatedly even after Henry was once more ruling in his own name. This is, however, a fear that was simply concerned with the nature of mental illness in itself and not with any stigma attached to it or any failure to understand. In itself, nobody openly doubted Henry's ability to rule once he had regained consciousness.

If this would ever be the case was, of course, unknown in the autumn of 1453, and a regent had to be found, which pitted factions at court against each other, much as factions at court had been working against each other during Henry's infancy and childhood. With Richard, Duke of York, becoming aware of the nature of Henry's illness, the cat was out of the bag and soon the general population became aware of it as well. There does not seem to have been any bulletin informing the population at large, as there was with physical illnesses. But then as now, there is no keeping a secret once a significant part of the population knows, as would have been the case once the nobility were aware. Of course, the nobility was only a very small part of the population, but nobles knowing also meant that their households, including lower-born servants knew, who would have also shared this, thus making the news spread like wildfire. Even if they had not been aware, it would have eventually been hard, if not outright impossible, to hide the turmoil of the government from the population at large. After all, government decisions would no longer have been made by Henry VI himself but in Henry's name, and while there was less news about such decisions available for the general population, news of this would still have seeped out, and indeed it did.

In fact, the chronicles about the world at large finding out about Henry's illness make for fascinating reading for those interested less in the solely political angle but in the reception and understanding of mental health issues. As has been mentioned above, in most cases the illness itself was treated no differently to a physical illness, as something considered unfortunate but that could not be helped and a cross that not only Henry, but also the country would have to bear. However, there was a fear expressed that would not have existed had Henry's illness been purely physical: a fear of ridicule and attack.[292]

This was not an entirely baseless fear, for after all there were many countries in Europe who were not exactly on the best of terms with England and Henry VI, for whom his incapacity was a gift. These would not hesitate to not only ridicule the country but use its momentary weakness in the absence of strong guidance by the king to attack the country, or at the very least, push through their own interests while disadvantaging England. It stands to reason that this is the main motive why the nature of Henry's illness was kept quiet for as long as possible, even more so than keeping the news from the nobility to stop them from fighting. As it happens, in fact, while in-fighting amongst the nobility could be a danger to the country, for the exact same reasons that Henry's illness could also be, signalling weakness to other countries and opening England up to ridicule and strong diplomatic disadvantage, a united nobility was of no use if the king's illness achieved these unhappy results on his own.

We have to remember that we do not know why the decision to keep Henry's mental incapacity from everyone for as long as possible was made. We can only guess. What we do know is that it would not have been done solely because mental illness in itself was considered bad. Nor would the reason have been that those suffering with them were shunned. There was a very recent precedent in Europe with Charles VI, Henry's own grandfather, and as such it was hardly unheard of or something that would make the whole country an outcast, the way some later historians have suggested.[293] Kings and queens were usually forgiven for many things that commoners or even the nobility would not be forgiven. So even if (which was not the case) those suffering from mental illness were routinely shunned by society, there needed to be no fear Henry would be, and therefore the reasons for keeping the nature of his illness quiet for so long must have been political. This is supported by the fact that the queen and her then closest advisor, the Duke of Somerset, were informed of the illness and passed off their reign as in the king's name[294] — in itself a dangerous choice, as Somerset was a rather controversial figure.[295] Had it been purely to keep up appearances and stop rumours about Henry's condition, it would not have been a smart move.

Even so, everyone must have known that it was unlikely that diplomatic relations could long continue without other countries knowing. Being kept in suspense for long, with all that was known was that the king was unable to receive visitors or act as king, would signal to those hostile to England or its king that there was something amiss, a weakness to be exploited. This could have been explained away if the nature of Henry's illness were openly announced as a physical illness that was serious, but he would soon recover from, like Edward IV did in 1463. Even so, without any confirmation such as Edward offered then, speculation would have doubtlessly continued.

Speculation about a monarch's health was not a new thing; lies and deception about the king or queen's state of health had precedent. In fact, in some cases even the king's death was kept a secret for some days, not just in England but in other countries as well. The most recent case, before Henry VI's mental illness, was Charles VI's — the extent of his illness kept from all but those closest to him. This explains, why rumours were circulating when Henry VI became ill, and which may be why Richard, Duke of York, acted as he did by insisting to see his cousin. After all, he must have been aware that there was a precedent for not always divulging the truth where a royal illness was concerned.[296]

In fact, despite Henry's history and his grandfather's history, there is actually no hint that anyone thought that Henry VI was suffering from a mental illness, or that this was the reason for him not showing himself.[297] This is sometimes assumed to have been the first thought, but this is pure hindsight. Even in the absence of evidence, there would be no reason to assume this would have been the first thought on everyone's mind. Since we do have evidence, we know it was not what was first feared. Mental illness was not a commonly discussed matter among non-medical professionals, and hence something that was very easily and readily suspected. As has been pointed out, even the accusation used as slander was not a common way to slander someone, and though there were accusations of Henry being simple-minded, or a 'fool', before 1450, it does not seem anyone actually expected him to become mentally ill before his mind gave way and he became catatonic.

As a matter of fact, this is rather interesting in itself, as Henry VI was not overly popular, though through no fault of his own. There were those who did not think he should be on the English throne; not because of any character failings of his own, but because of how he had inherited it — his grandfather, Henry IV, had usurped the throne from the childless Richard II. Though that had been over twenty years ago, when the infant Henry VI came to the throne it was far from forgotten. There had been rebellions for that reason against Henry IV and even Henry VI's father, Henry V. There were never any against Henry VI because of this until the mid-1450s, but we do know from evidence that it was remembered, and there were still those who kept closely in mind that he should not have been on the throne had the actual line of succession been followed.

This was part of why many sources considered Richard, Duke of York's actions when Henry was incapacitated rather problematic: not because of any worry about illness, about Henry being dead even, and least of all because of mental illness. This was not the focus when the Duke of York's actions in August 1453 and afterwards were addressed contemporarily. The problem with his actions, the problem with him in particular knowing that Henry was unable to rule for himself was that, by rights of inheritance from Richard II, Richard, Duke of York, had a far bigger claim to the English throne than anyone else, including Henry VI himself.[298]

What exactly it was that made Henry unable to rule was therefore irrelevant; what mattered was that he could not rule, period. The reasons were only considered important to contemporary sources such as *The English Chronicle*[299] and *Whethamsted's Register*[300] to understand whether or not Henry would recover soon and how big his chances were to rule again.

The chances of him being cured, and his contemporaries' understanding of this, is a subject that will be addressed later. For the purposes of this chapter, all that is important is that there were different opinions on it and therefore the illness was received with differing degrees of worry, as were Richard, Duke of York's actions.

Even so, as pointed out above, there is actually no reason whatsoever to assume that mental illness was something that was expected to strike Henry VI down in August 1453, nor anything that was ever used politically against him. Henry was not a particularly popular king, and by 1453 had gone through several strong crises, the last of which was not yet a year ago, when he became catatonic in August of that year.

In fact, it has sometimes been thought to have been a cause for Henry's mental illness that his supposedly already feeble mind gave way under the stress of the years immediately before his illness hit. This theory, occasionally alluded to in contemporary fifteenth-century sources, is one that has become especially favoured in the last few decades, since the understanding of post-traumatic stress disorder (PTSD) has come on leaps and bounds. Henry VI had indeed had a rather trying time before he became catatonic in 1453, even for the fifteenth century, and even for a fifteenth-century king. Not only had he lost several people close to him, such as two of his uncles who had acted as protectors for him during his childhood, but he had lost them under very difficult circumstances.

In a manner of speaking, Henry's troubles, and, some historians assert, his trouble with mental health, started with the loss of his uncle Humphrey, Duke of Gloucester, who died shortly before he could stand trial for treason against Henry. Humphrey's story has been told elsewhere in detail, and it is not the aim of this book to rehash it. However, for an understanding of mental health, his downfall is somewhat important, as it has sometimes been used as an indicator that Henry VI first showed symptoms of his mental health failing at that time, and that in fact, the Duke of Gloucester's fate is a good example for it.

Humphrey, Duke of Gloucester, had lost most of his political, if not popular, significance before his death in 1447, with his wife being accused of treason, but even so, he had not been shy about stating his opinion all throughout the 1440s. Most of his opinions were opposed to the policies Henry VI was pursuing, from the way he wished the war in France to end to his choice of wife and queen. However, he had never actually been treasonous, and it was considered at the time that the charges against him were trumped up.[301]

Since direct criticism of the king was not really possible at the time, and since Henry was thought to be a meek and easily led man, this accusation was not laid against him, but instead against several of his closest advisors. Most notable of these was William, Duke of Suffolk, who had been politically very opposed to the Duke of Gloucester.[302] However, after Henry VI went mad, there were voices who considered the fact he accused his uncle, who had served him well and been correct with many of his predictions as to political life, as a sign of his madness.[303] This is hardly far-fetched and would hold up even to modern ideas of mental illness: Henry could indeed have been gripped by paranoia, encouraged by others or not, and considered the Duke of Gloucester's statements against his chosen course of political action as threats against his person. As has been pointed out, the same can be said for several events Henry VI gave orders for, which have traditionally been assigned to his wife, his advisors, anyone but him.

Even if Humphrey, Duke of Gloucester's charge of treason had actually been brought by one of his political enemies, not his nephew himself, and even if his death, as evidence indicates, was just a sad coincidence at the time it happened, it must still have been a blow for Henry VI. Even if he did not personally mourn his uncle, the Duke of Gloucester's death meant a lot of political upheaval against him, for the first time against him personally as well. Henry VI had never been a particularly popular man, but until 1447, criticism against his government had rarely, if ever, been directed against him personally.[304] As such, it would doubtlessly have been a painful experience for him to suddenly find himself reviled by parts of the population, but hardly an unusual one for any mediaeval king. In itself, it would not have been considered, at the time or afterwards, to have made Henry VI's mind crack.

However, the very fact that Henry VI reacted politically unwisely to this criticism meant the situation only became worse. His continued favour of William, Duke of Suffolk, a man who has often been assumed, probably correctly, to have acted as a father figure to Henry VI during his adolescent and early adult years, led to downright viral hatred against the man. By 1450, this hatred forced Henry to take him prisoner as he, too, was charged with treason.[305]

Henry VI managed to see him acquitted for that, but it came at the price of having Suffolk banished for five years. This did not save the unfortunate duke, and he was beheaded as he made his way into exile. This crime saw Henry faced with the realisation of the personal side of bad kingship, and, following hot on its heels, with a rebellion.[306] Henry sent men to crush the rebels, but the matter was not finished with that. Rumours circulated that Suffolk's death had been ordered and even, in fact, that the extreme hatred against the man was caused by Henry VI's own distant cousin and heir presumptive, Richard, Duke of York. There were even rumours of Richard being one of the leading minds behind the rebellion shortly after Suffolk's death.[307]

Henry refused to accept this as a possibility,[308] though his queen certainly did entertain the thought.[309] However, he could not close his eyes to what happened shortly afterwards, when the Duke of York actually *did* move against his government. As the Duke of York was a smart man who did not want to be executed for treason, he stressed his loyalty to the king and that he only wanted to free him from his bad advisors. The same claim had been made by the rebels of 1450, and it was a staple of political rebels in the Middle Ages.

Henry VI was lucky in that he still had enough support and the Duke of York's rebellion failed in late 1452,[310] but when he went mad in 1453, there were voices connecting the events of the last six or so years with his breakdown.[311] It is possible that this was at least partly what happened, but the scant evidence we have does not actually support this. On the contrary, while Henry VI was usually a meek man and noted to be so,[312] he had been rather harsh and cruel to rebels in the last few years and had managed to put his foot down several times.[313]

This, too, has sometimes been taken as a sign of his mental illness, but it is a modern understanding. Contemporarily, if his situation was blamed at all, it was more the fact that all these traumatising events had happened and not Henry's reaction to it all. This, too, is rather illuminating not only for Henry's case in itself and his own mental state and the exploration of his mental illness, but also for the perception of the understanding of mental illness as a whole in fifteenth-century England. In short, there was some understanding of the effects traumatic events such as brutal losses and betrayals can have on the human psyche. Though there was no name for it at the time, and long afterward, this was suggested when *Whethamsted's Register* said that Henry 'did not cultivate the art of war'[314] and that this was why '[a] disease and disorder of such a sort overcame the king that he lost his wits and memory for a time, and nearly all his body was so uncoordinated and out of control that he could neither walk, nor hold his head upright, nor easily move from where he sat'.[315] In modern terms, the suggestion was that Henry suffered from post-traumatic stress disorder.

Especially for modern readers with a better understanding of mental health problems and the cause and effect of mental illnesses, this sounds fairly plausible, which is presumably the reason why this theory has become more popular in the last few decades. However, it is a theory that has two big problems: being catatonic is not a common symptom of PTSD, and moreover, there is no evidence of Henry suffering from it.

Henry had shown no signs of this disorder at any point in his life, or even in the years leading up to his catatonia. The symptoms are flashbacks, night terrors and physical symptoms such as nausea and shakiness[316] and while until very recently, they would have been considered shameful and Henry VI would have doubtlessly gone to all trouble to hide them, there is absolutely no way he could have hidden them completely. Even if he had, by some miracle, been able to do so before his mental illness either started in 1453 or became common knowledge after it had become so drastic, after that happened there would have been stories about it. The very fact that there was never anything of the sort even suggested is a silence that is loud and clear. As much as anyone can say, so long after the fact, though the stress he suffered from may very well have played into his mental breakdown, Henry VI did not suffer from PTSD. That this is still suggested makes it clear that the concept was one that was known and understood at the time, but one that was not well known enough to make any distinction from other illnesses.

In fact, there is something else notable about Henry VI, his mental health, his mental illness and the perception thereof both of his nobles and the population at large: though both contemporaries and centuries' worth of historians have analysed Henry's reign for traces of behaviour indicating mental ill-health before he became catatonic in 1453, there were few suggestions made of Henry being mentally ill, with only some comments being made by commoners to suggest he was 'a natural fool'.[317] Though this could indicate that those in power simply wished to avoid making such an accusation, for political or personal reasons, this is unlikely in the light of the fact that even at the height of his unpopularity in 1450, with some poems being circulated and mocking songs sung by rebels, which outright attacked Henry, even threatening his throne, there was no allusion made to him being in any way mad or not completely mentally healthy.[318]

Once more, there are several conclusions that can be drawn from this. First, it means that mental illness was not as much of a slander as other accusations were, and being connected with it was not actually seen as the mark of shame it is often claimed to have been. If so, there would have been allusions made to it. Even if Henry VI had been possessed of the sturdiest mental health, the very fact that his French grandfather had been mentally ill could have been used against him. That this was not done was not because it was considered of no consequence — his grandfather having nothing to do with him — as his ancestry actually was used against him. The fact his mother had been French and he himself was therefore half-French was used against him repeatedly,[319] both during the 1450 rebellion and the lead-up to it as well as in the years before. If it had been in any way a political advantage to tie Henry to his grandfather's mental illness, it would have been done. That it was not obviously shows there would have been no gain from it, neither politically nor in any populistic way, to make Henry more unpopular. It was only after Henry VI became openly mentally ill that the connection was made, and then it was more often used as an explanation rather than as an accusation or anything of the sort.

In fact, contrary to what is often claimed, the many political criticisms of Henry VI and his politics as well as his behaviour before 1453 was never actually tied to any expectation, assumption or idea of him being less than mentally perfectly healthy, though later, it was sometimes used as an explanation. None of the language suggests that anyone thought he was anything but simply politically singularly inept, and uninterested in the business of kingship. There could actually be a case made that his mental illness overshadows the rest of his personality,[320] not even primarily in contemporary sources but mainly in scholarly work. Most of Henry's failures as a mediaeval king are explained by this mental illness, in a way they were distinctly not when they actually happened.

The most blatant example of this is Henry's reported kindness, gentleness and lack of interest in kingship. Most modern works seem to at the very least imply that this was due to his mental illness, such as Ralph Alan Griffiths and Lauren Johnson.[321] Some go farther than that and state that was the case, an example for this being Matthew Lewis in his biography of Richard, Duke of York.[322] However, nobody at the time thought so, not even after his mental illness became widely known. The viewpoint taken by Henry's contemporaries, or at the least the only viewpoint recorded to have been taken by Henry's contemporaries, was simply that his personality was singularly unsuited for kingship, but not that this was in any way linked to any mental illness or lack of mental sturdiness. In many cases, it was not even seen as a character flaw. On the contrary, it was often considered as a sign of his actual kindness, a generally good trait, simply badly suited to a king.

A good example of this viewpoint is found in the contemporary source written by John Blacman, which says that Henry was a kind, pious man whose religious visions made him, in effect, too good to be a king.[323] In fact, an idea that was often repeated was that Henry VI would have been better suited to life as a monk,[324] a life that was at least idealised as being calm, devoted to God and good deeds, though this was not always what actually happened. That this was an assessment that was probably correct can be seen in Henry's actions and successes as king. He was interested in architecture, in the Church and in scholarship, and used his powers as king to foster and promote this.

This was simply seen as having the wrong character to be king, not as a sign that something was wrong with him, much less that he was actually mentally ill. Nor was it regarded so after he became catatonic in 1453 and his reputation quickly shifted from gentle but ineffectual king to him being 'the mad king'.[325] Even then, his achievements, such as they were, were not dismissed, or in fact his character analysed as having been entirely influenced by the mental illness he sadly suffered from.

On the contrary. If anything, his gentle character was seen as being the cause of his mental illness, as it meant that kingship was simply not suited for him. As mentioned above, there was actually no accusation against Henry in this way, any more than there was any accusation against William, Viscount Beaumont, in the idea that his character was unsuited to him being an active participant in a civil war. While his mental illness and his character, which actually was very unsuited to mediaeval kingship, limited his success as a king, there was no dismissal of him as a king entirely, much less as a person. Several modern historians have not awarded Henry the same respect, with one describing Henry VI as an 'utterly useless muppet'.[326]

Keeping this in mind, Henry VI's contemporaries were actually fairly kind to him, especially by comparison. Perhaps most importantly, they did not, even after they knew of his mental illness, consider his medical history to be the sum of all Henry ever was, or even to have influenced all his actions.[327] Nor do they ever actually blame Henry for being mentally ill, even when using the fact he suffered from it politically against him.

In fact, while the knowledge of this mental illness was one that did change the perception of Henry VI, his character and his kingship in some ways, this was not considered as important as is usually assumed in history books. This can be seen in many primary sources such as the *Whethamsted Chronicle*, which details that even after Henry recovered, his actions were not generally judged by his illness, or his opinion and actions invalidated because of it.

This will be detailed more closely, but there is another point that needs to be made first: the fact that this fairly gentle behaviour towards Henry VI was not just a solely English phenomenon. While many foreign rulers and their governments tried to use it for their own gain and to disadvantage Henry VI and his government, there is absolutely no suggestion that this was done due to any maliciousness towards Henry himself, or even due to a dislike of mental illness and a wish to see someone who had it ostracised.

In fact, somewhat strangely, there was not even any reference made in foreign sources, such as French, Burgundian or Flemish ones, that this was thought of as a punishment from God. This is a point not often addressed when the political implications of Henry VI's mental illness are examined, though it is certainly a point of interest. Since the late Middle Ages were a very religious age, often any difficulties in any area of life were seen as interference by God, either as a cross someone would have to bear or a punishment of some sort. The religious ramifications will be discussed more below; for the point made in this chapter, it is simply worth noting that there was actually no argument made that invoked God or used Henry's mental health issues as some sort of statement by God.

From a modern perspective, the point could be made that this was either out of decency, a wish not to attack a mentally ill man, which would, however, presuppose a gentleness towards mentally ill people not usually associated with the Middle Ages, or else a fear of causing such punishment by commenting on it. However, if so, it would differ very much from how other misfortunes happening to kings or countries, or even how other illnesses were treated. When, some thirty years after Henry VI's mental illness became known, Edward IV died at the age of only 40, leaving behind a young son who was thought to inherit the throne,

French sources did not hesitate to gloat about this, stating the sickness that had suddenly killed him to be a result of his failure at diplomacy with their own government.[328] This was not the only such case; in fact, often when two countries were hostile to one another and a misfortune befell one of the monarchs of these countries, there would be at the very least some veiled comments as to it being God's punishment or a sign of who was favoured by God and which side would win. Examples for this were the sudden death of the unfortunate Charles VI,[329] and conversely, also the sudden death of Henry V only weeks before that.[330] Obviously, such political point scoring extended to the sudden death of a monarch as well as to physical illness suffered by one, as seen by what happened after Edward IV's sickness and death.

The failure to do it in Henry VI's case is rather inexplicable and there are no documents to shine any light on it, so that we can only speculate as to why this was. Perhaps the most likely explanation is that mental illness was far more an unchartered territory than physical illness was, and as such, any message from God would have been far more vague than one for a physical illness, or even one for the king's sudden death — in short, easily explicable and understandable tragedies. This would have been even more so since the symptoms of Henry VI's mental illness seem to have fairly baffled his physicians. Nor would physicians in another country, most notably France, have had any more of an idea as to what this showed about the illness he actually suffered from and, perhaps more importantly, what it said about his chances of recovery. In fact, it is possible that nobody was even quite sure what it meant for the future and, therefore, what sort of message from God it could even be. It stands to reason that this was why no such comments were made, at least initially, though why none were made after Henry had been suffering from catatonia for over a year and the hopes of him recovering were starting to be considered slim is something that must remain a mystery forever.

Perhaps, the reality of dealing with Henry's illness and working around it was one that became so important that there was little to no time to consider if his illness was good or bad for his country as well as other European countries. Certainly, by the time France and other neighbouring countries had found out about what had happened to Henry VI and the state of the English government, a solution, if a temporary one, had been found. This is logical; no one in the English government would have wanted to risk such important and potentially dangerous information to be passed on before a solution had been found, even if different parties disagreed on what this solution should be.

There are ways that the foreign nobility and foreign governments could have found out about Henry's illness before it became widely known, or before it was officially treated as fact in foreign diplomacy by the government acting in Henry's name. In fact, this is almost certainly what happened; like the English nobility, the French and Burgundian nobility at the very least would have had spies at the English court, to tell them, if not exact news, at the very least the gossip that was circulating. After it was known to the English nobility, there would have been no possibility to keep a lid on the news, of course. Just as it would have seeped out to the English population, it would have also become known in foreign countries. This is quite logical and there would have been no need for any malicious intent; then as now, gossip did spread, and so it would have in this case.

Simply, Henry's illness in itself was treated with a lot of respect, with no snide comments against him at all.[331] This was true even after Henry VI, who was, for the time being, treated as if he was an infant again, had been given a lord protector in the person of Richard, Duke of York, and his government had taken up work again, in his name rather than with him being the leading figure, the ruler. This work would have included diplomatic relations with other countries. It would have been through these relations that France, Burgundy, Spain and the other European countries would have been officially informed of Henry's mental illness.

We do not actually know with what words Henry VI's mental illness was explained, though it stands to reason that Richard, Duke of York and his regency council would have seen to it that it was presented to the foreign dignitaries, probably ambassadors, in the least damaging way possible and given an explanation to these men that put the best possible spin on the situation.

Sadly, we cannot know what this explanation was, but we do have some ambassadors' reports from that time, which give us an idea and especially tell us how it was received. There is no mention made about Henry's catatonia in any of the documents on foreign policies we have.

The fact that all ambassador reports all but ignored Henry's sickness suggests that there was an effort made to hide this illness. This is not very strange, but it is strange that no side rumour, nor otherwise hostile report survives by any of the foreign commentators.

Once more, this dryness is very telling as to how mental illness was viewed at the time. At least at this high level of society, there is no indication of any resentment or refusal to associate with it, and absolutely no blame given to the person suffering from the mental illness, and that the difficulties seen arising from it were purely political. At most, there was unrecorded mockery in private. Even if so, though, it would mean that though there was prejudice and some sort of resentment against those mentally ill, it was, at least for those so high-born private and not actually systemic. (Though as discussed above, this was different if the person suffering from mental illness was not a king or a high-ranking noble, or even if the king or high-ranking noble was suffering from a more violent form of mental illness.)

It must have helped that Henry VI's mental illness incapacitated him entirely. Though particularly horrible for him, there is a suggestion it stopped both the flow of rumours before the nature of his illness was known, and also the prejudice when it was known. This is actually fairly logical; as shall be seen below, mediaeval conceptions of mental health and mental illnesses were not exactly the same as ours. While, as has been pointed out in Chapter 2, there was a lot of overlap, especially in the considered way causes of such illnesses were treated which was much more advanced than we today give the people living in the Middle Ages credit for. But their ideas of what mental illness actually looked like was somewhat different.[332]

In a way, of course, this too has to be differentiated. Quite obviously, as can be seen from the varied entries found in the coroner's rolls,[333] quoted and discussed in Chapter 1, there was at least an awareness that mental illness could manifest in a variety of symptoms. Even so, the most common association, the association echoed in contemporary literature and also in art and even mediaeval plays was that of the so-called raving lunatic, a man or woman walking around the streets, waving and gesticulating, talking to thin air, being convinced they were surrounded by people who are not actually there. A variation of that was that this 'raving lunatic' thought he or she was being followed by someone or something that was not there.

This sort of mental illness, somewhat echoing the symptoms of Charles VI and therefore being widely known all over Europe at least in the fifteenth century was hard, if not impossible, to hide. While the person suffering from it could be stopped from walking around, as indeed

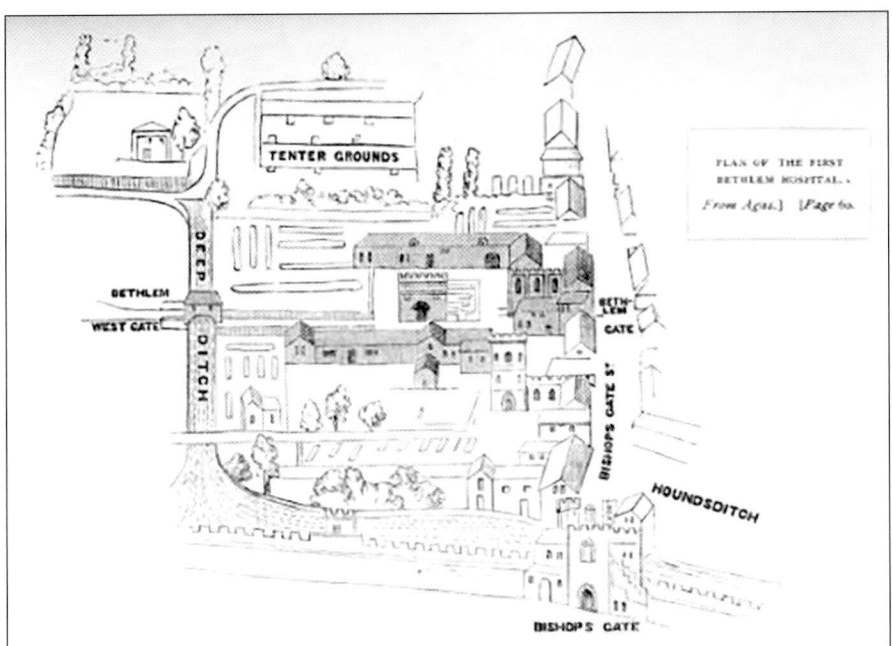

Ground plan of Bedlam (Bethlem) Hospital. (From *Chapters in the History of the Insane* by Daniel Hack Tuke, p.61, published 1882. Public domain.) This ground plan is not a contemporary one, but based on architectural research. It shows the approximate arrangement of the hospital as well as its size.

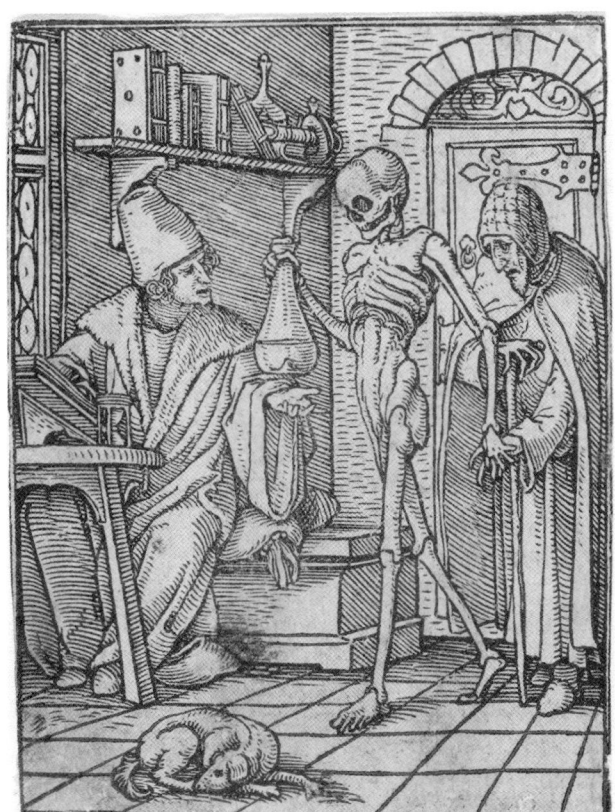

The Physician, 1526. (Hans Lützelburger, Hans Holbein der Jüngere. Held by the National Portrait Gallery. Public domain.) A depiction of a physician performing his job while battling a very visible death. The vial held by death could contain some sort of bodily fluid, which was often used in mediaeval medicine.

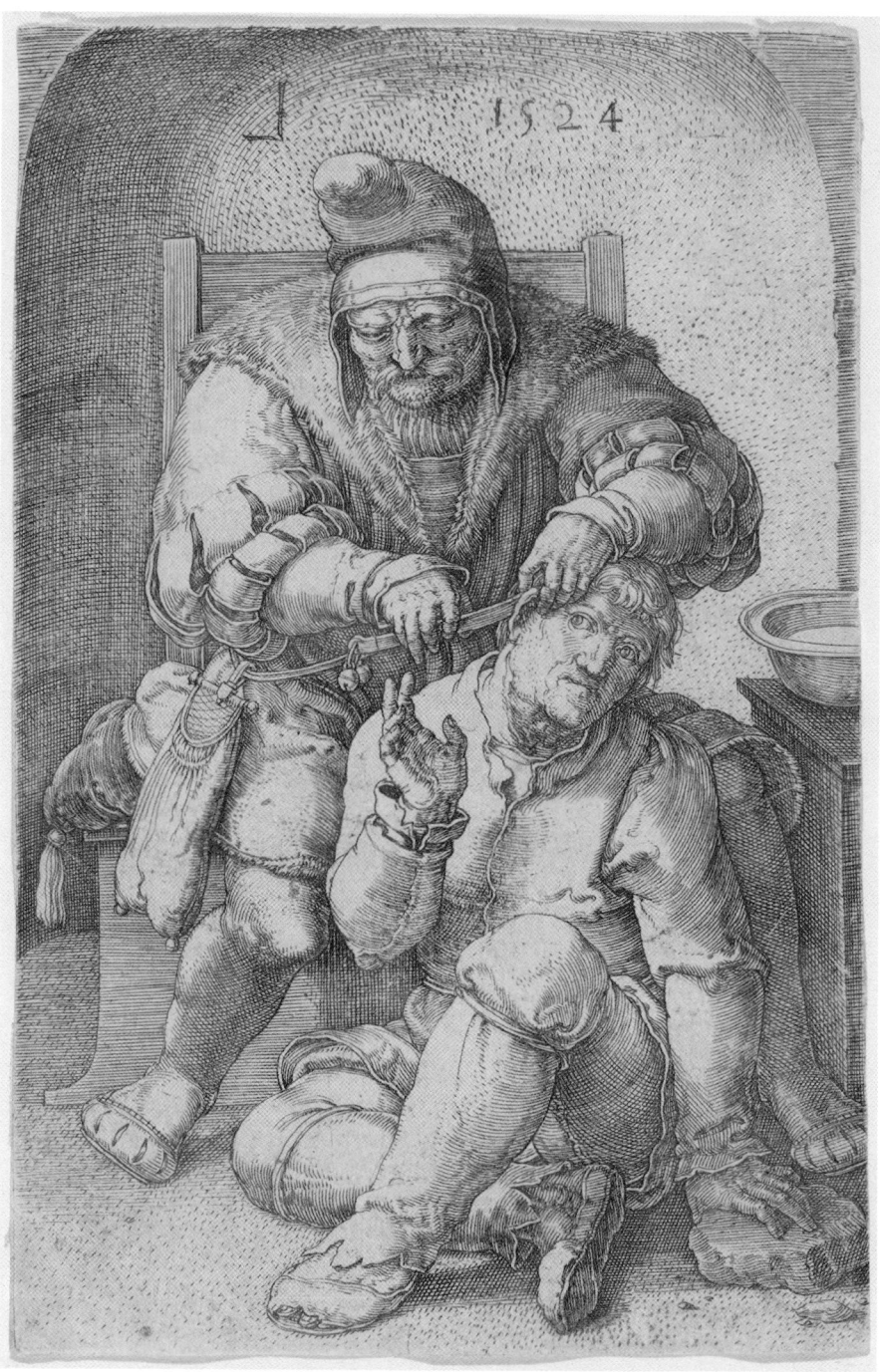

The Surgeon, 1524. (Lukas van Leyden. Held by the National Portrait Gallery. Public domain.) A depiction of a surgeon performing a procedure on a patient. Though there is no hint given to what sort of procedure it is meant to be, treatments given by surgeons to both the physically and mentally ill often resembled each other. This picture, therefore, shows an idealised version of a procedure that many mentally ill people would have undergone.

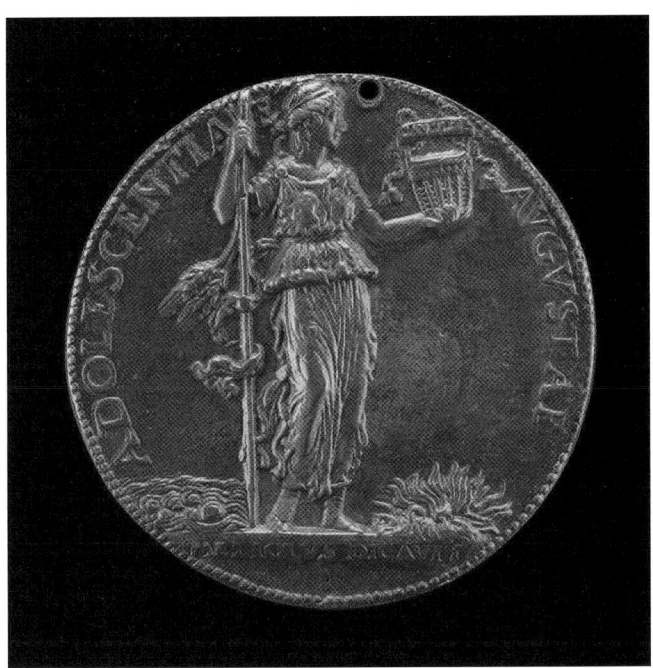

Health/Prudence Standing Between Sea and Fire, c.1480. (Bartolomeo Melioli. Held by the National Portrait Gallery. Public domain.) This picture is sometimes rendered as a personification of health and sometimes as a personification of prudence. It gives an interesting idea of late mediaeval views on life, and that virtues as well as physical and mental wellbeing were beleaguered by dangers from all sides.

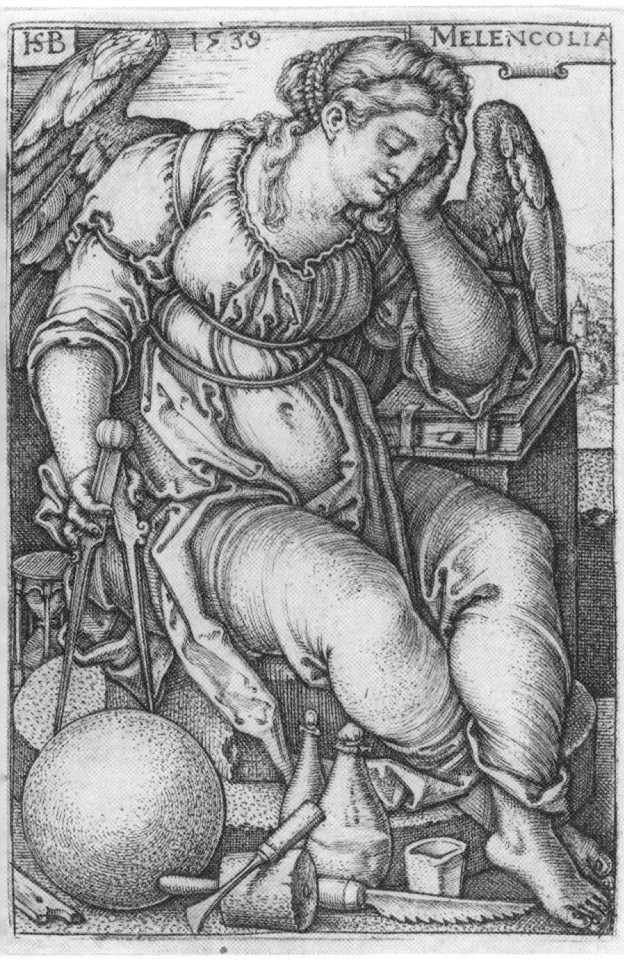

Melancholia, 1539. (Sebald Beham. Held by the National Portrait Gallery. Public domain.) A personification of melancholy – depression in modern terms. Interestingly, it shows the person suffering from many symptoms that even today are still associated with depression, such as her being surrounded by chaos and being unable to do anything about it, and clearly having no interest in any of her surroundings.

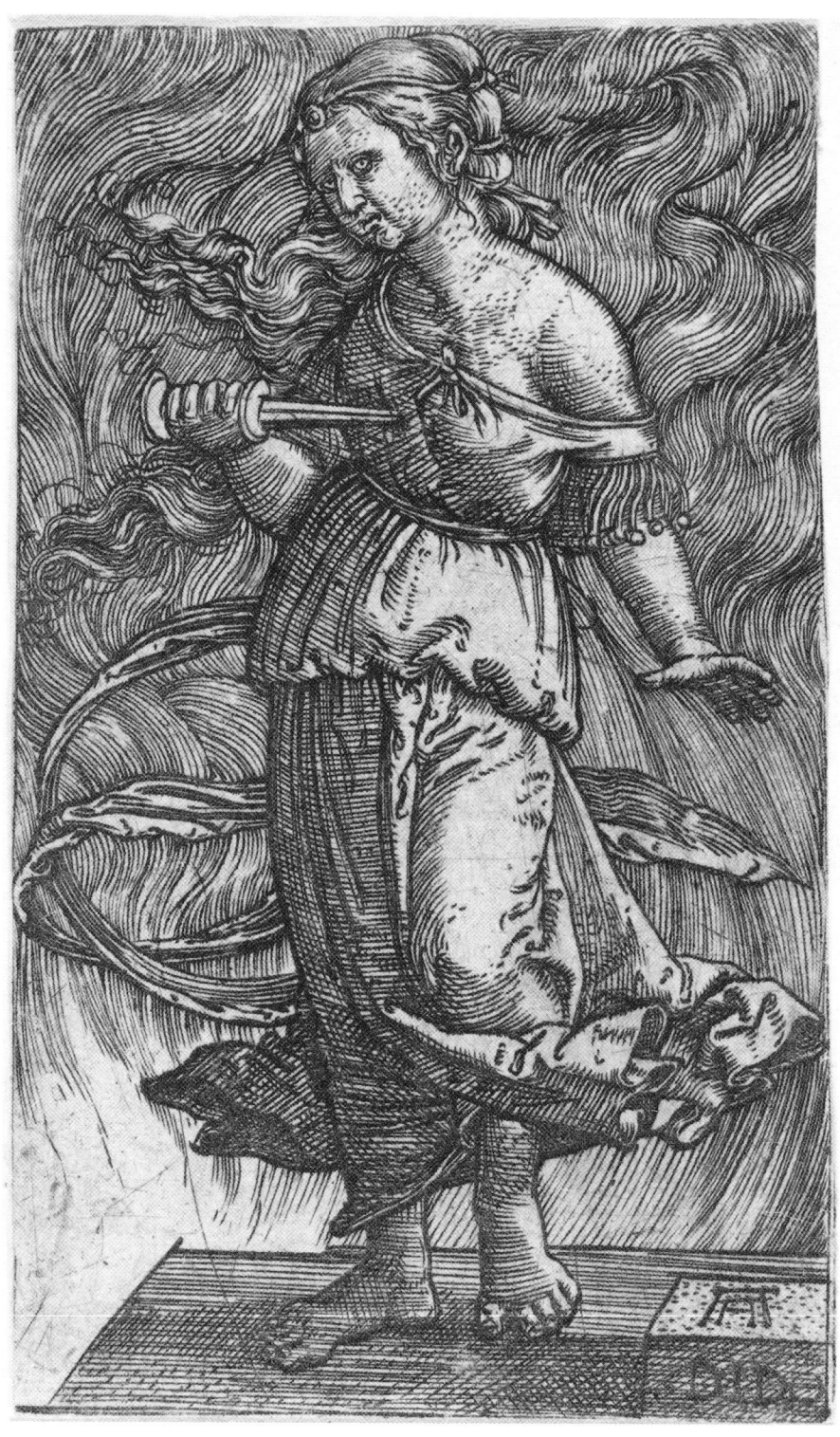

Dido, *c.*1520. (Sebald Beham. Held by the National Portrait Gallery. Public domain.) The artistic choices echo that of Altdorfer's picture opposite.

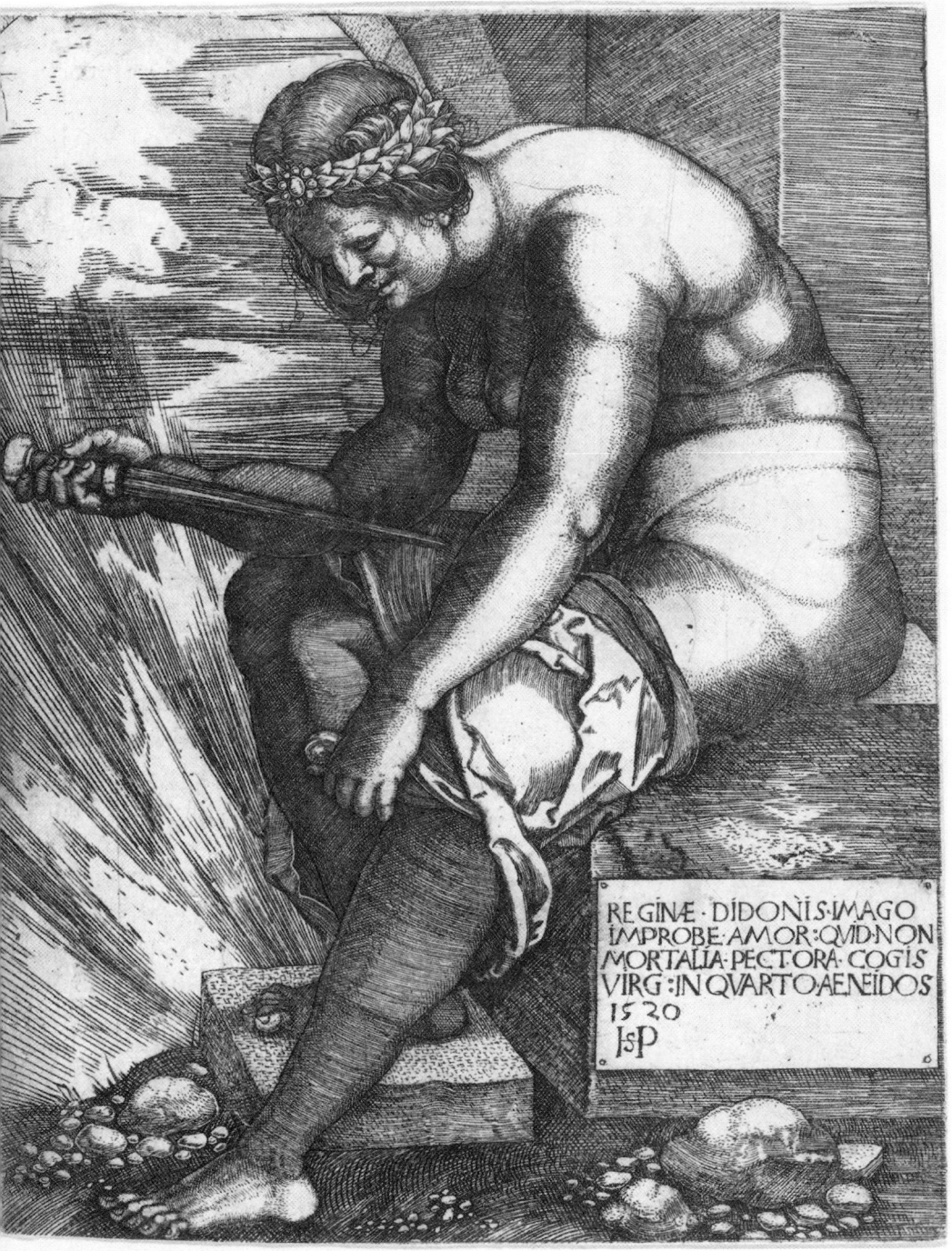

The Suicide of Dido, c.1500. (Albrecht Altdorfer. Held by the National Portrait Gallery. Public domain.) Another late mediaeval depiction of a famous mythological suicide. Doubtlessly, the fact the subject is naked is partly simply an artistic choice by the male artist, but it is a common choice in the depiction of suicides, both male and female. As such, it also reflects the idea that those committing suicide were completely distant from all social rules.

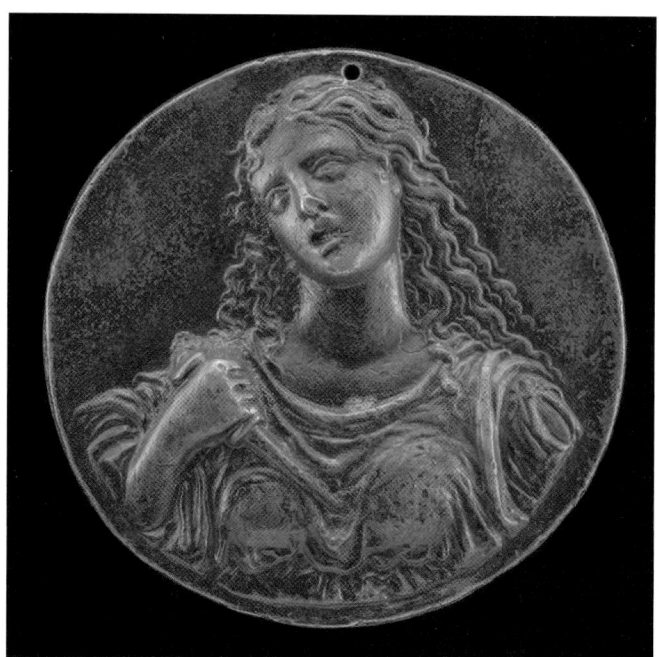

Lucretia Stabbing Herself, late fifteenth/early sixteenth century. (Moderno. Held by the National Portrait Gallery. Public domain.) Another famous mythological suicide. It is interesting that many artistic choices, including the weapon, echo that of most depictions of the suicide of Dido. There is something of an underlying suggestion that suicides were caused and executed in a similar way. Deaths from other causes resembling each other were also portrayed in the same fashion.

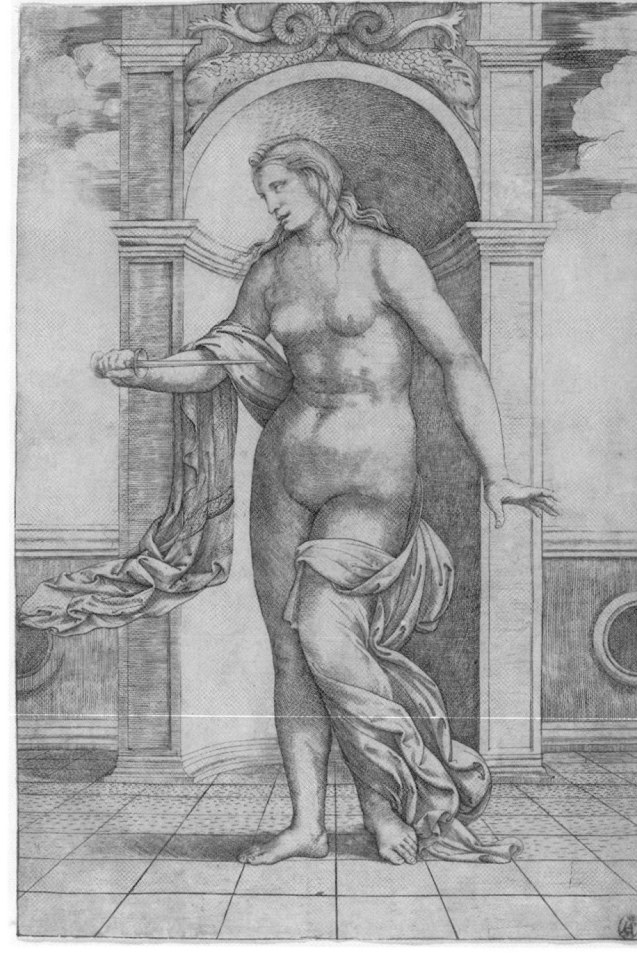

*Lucretia, c.*1510. (Jacopo Francia. Held by the National Portrait Gallery. Public domain.) Another depiction of Lucretia's suicide. Mythical stories, and especially mythical deaths, were a fertile subject for late mediaeval paintings. There is something of a religious aspect in that too, portraying non-Christian figures committing acts and/or dying deaths that were believed to cause damnation. Conversely, pictures like this one of Lucretia do not show any distaste, and so by choosing these subjects painters could show such deaths in a compassionate light.

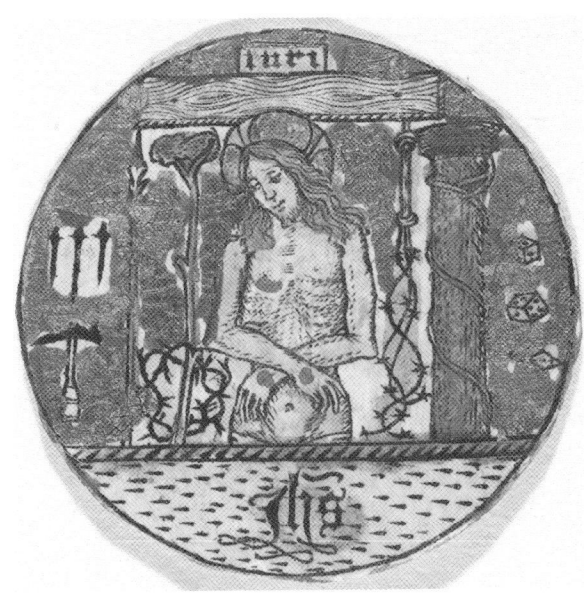

Christ as the Man of Sorrows, c.1450/1460. (Anonymous. Held by the National Portrait Gallery. Public domain.) A very popular choice of artistic representation of Jesus Christ in the Middle Ages. Rather than him being shown as solely divine, he is shown as a man suffering. The title is based on a passage from the Bible, describing Christ's suffering by saying he was at the time 'a man rejected and despised'. It was therefore often used as a comfort for those rejected and despised by society, as those suffering from mental illness sometimes were. This was a connection often made.

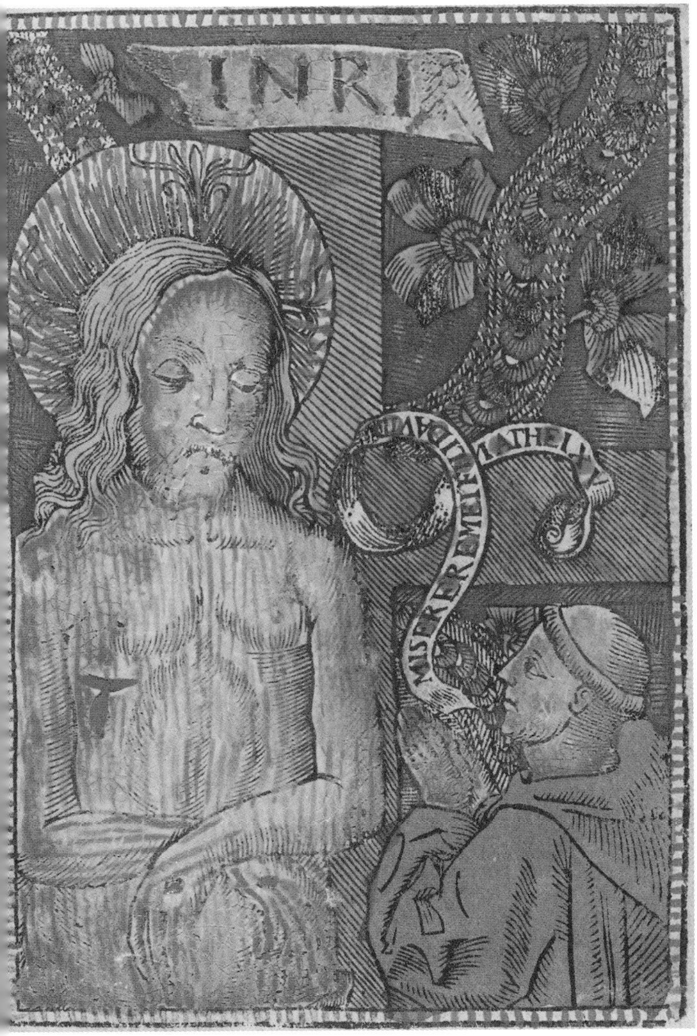

The Man of Sorrows with a Franciscan, c.1490/1500. (Anonymous. Held by the National Portrait Gallery. Public domain.) Another depiction of Jesus Christ as a man of sorrow, here curiously shown as both divine, halo clearly visible, and a human being suffering. The artist shows this version of Jesus Christ as just as important and just as praiseworthy as other depictions of him.

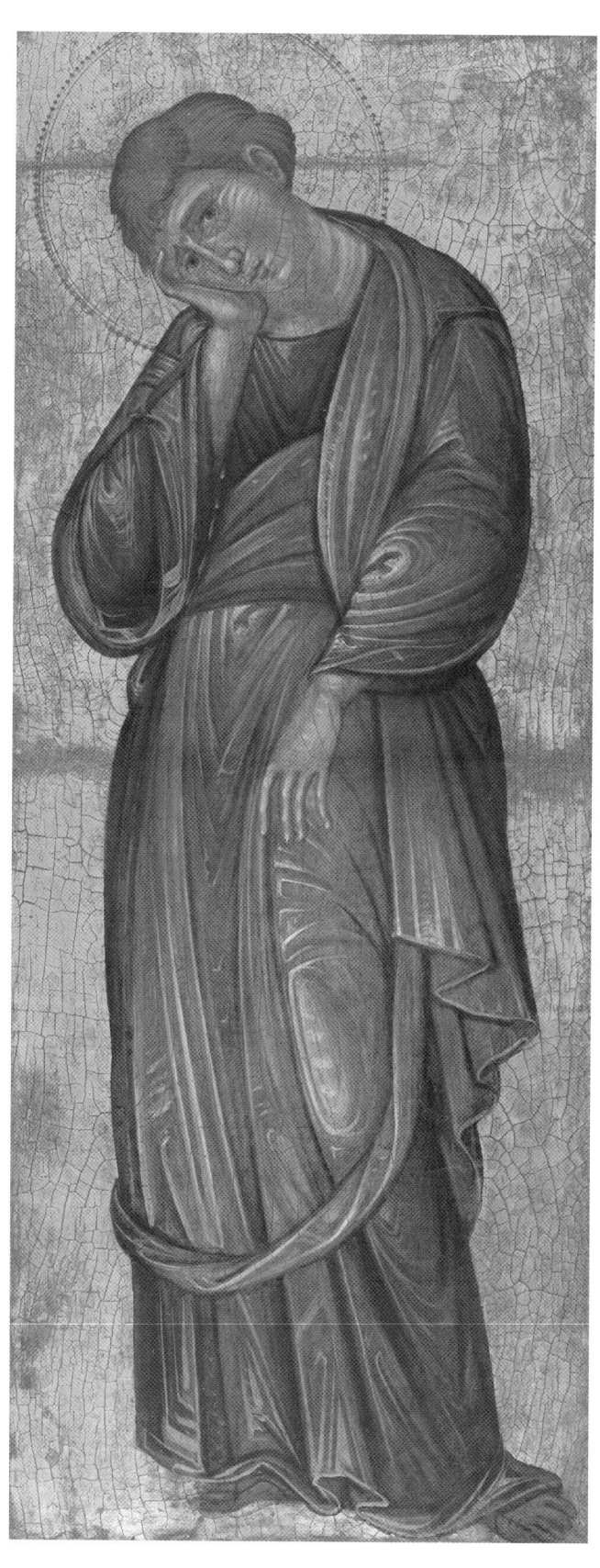

The Mourning Saint John the Evangelist, c.1270/1275. (Anonymous. Held by the National Portrait Gallery. Public domain.) A depiction of mourning, in excesses often seen as mental illness in medieval society. By showing saints as equally suffering from such emotions, it was made obvious that there was nothing shameful in it, and that it was only a part of being human.

Charles sometimes was,[334] it was a loud and rather obtrusive kind of illness, the symptoms of which would have immediately been passed on and given courtiers and servants at least a clue of what was happening.

Henry VI, notably, did not have this kind of illness at all. On the contrary, his illness manifested in him being catatonic and unable to recognise anybody, and unable to react to anything that was happening; an illness that could even have been physical, at least as long as physicians had not examined him to be able to tell it was not so.

In fact, there is an indication that this was the first assumption when Henry, suddenly and unexpectedly, fell ill. Though with our modern-day knowledge of mental illnesses, we can make assumptions as to what part of Henry's behaviour might in fact have been triggered by his mental illness, as opposed to decisions he made and behaviour he exhibited when sound of mind, there was none of that knowledge in his own day, and no interest in making such assumptions. Until he became ill in 1453, there is absolutely no indication whatsoever that anyone expected him to become mentally ill, much less actually considered him to be so.

Therefore, when Henry first became unresponsive, from what we know of the actions and treatments his physicians chose, there was an assumption that he was suffering from some sort of physical illness.[335] However, it soon became clear that his body, at the very least, was working well, in some rather gruesome treatments designed to find this out, which included 'head purges' and other blood-letting. In modern terms, they were designed to test if Henry was in a coma or was paralysed by some other physical ailment.[336] Only when these treatments had no effect, other than showing that there was no physical ailment, and that Henry moreover did not react to the treatments at all, did the realisation dawn that he was in the grips of some sort of mental illness.[337]

As such, there was less chance of information trickling down, to both the population and other, perhaps somewhat hostile, countries, such as France, before the official, governmentally sanctioned version was passed around. Even so, while this might be something of an explanation as to why there was less speculation about this illness than about most other illnesses afflicting monarchs, both mental and physical, it does not account for the kindness in dealing with them. The only explanation that makes sense is that nobody was really comfortable in doing so, and thus that there was a greater sensitivity about mental health and mental illness than seems suggested by language that is often actively discriminatory to modern ears.

Even so, it would have been absurdly naive to expect Henry VI's enemies not to seize the chance while he, and therefore his government, was weak to try and use this to their advantage. Again, this has nothing to do with the nature of mental illness or even the nature of the treatment of mental illness in the fifteenth century. It was simply politics: try and take any advantage that presented itself, worry not about the morals. The same would doubtlessly have been done had Henry VI been stricken with a physical illness or injury that was suspected or feared to make him unable to actively rule for a very long time, possibly forever. Despite the suggested connection between Henry's enemies gaining power at that time and discrimination against people suffering from mental illness, the evidence does not bear out such a connection.

In fact, the disadvantages suffered by Henry VI, and more concretely his country and government, were purely of a political nature. It is hard to see them as anything but an indirect result of Henry's incapacity, and unconnected to the exact nature of this incapacity. In fact, these were aims his enemies, both in his own government and abroad, had worked on for over several years: the French king succeeded in finally pressing his advantage and not only managing to get England to agree to a peace treaty that was advantageous to France and disadvantageous to England, he also managed to throw English forces out of France almost completely, with the only exception being the town of Calais,[338] which would remain in English hands for another hundred years. Though the English forces had been consistently losing to the French for twenty years by then, the end of the so-called Hundred Years' War is usually said to have been 1453, the moment that the English, due to Henry VI's insanity and the in-fighting that followed over how to try and win a losing war, stopped being able to fight in it.

As such, France could be seen as the greatest winner of the crisis caused by Henry VI's sudden mental illness, but they were hardly the only ones. There were others who used the advantage offered to them by Henry's illness, most notably his distant cousin Richard, Duke of York. As alluded to above, he had been locked in a power struggle with several of Henry's closest advisors for several years before Henry VI became catatonic, and had usually been on the losing side. However, he had some powerful supporters, was a well-liked figure and, moreover, was one of the highest-ranking and highest-born nobles. When Henry VI was taken out of the equation by his illness, Richard knew how to seize his chance and catapulted himself into a position of power and saw to it his enemies were far removed from it, even going so far as to see Edmund Beaufort, Duke of Somerset, locked in the Tower of London.[339]

This has often seen him labelled as an enemy of the king's, but the situation was not quite as easy and it would not be fair to paint him as callously happy about Henry's illness, much less using it to punish him. After all, while a rebel or malcontent stating that his problems were with the king's advisors rather than the king himself was normal and not actually revealing his actual feelings and intentions, Richard, Duke of York, showed no intention of wanting to unseat Henry VI until 1460.[340] Perhaps, more notably, he never once tried to use his mental illness against him. Even when he did finally claim the throne, he did not mention Henry's mental illness at all as reason as to why he was unsuitable for the task of being king.[341]

This is the final point of interest in Henry VI's fascinating case and its significance to mediaeval understanding: the utter lack of using his mental illness as slander, or even as a reason as to why he should not be king and was unsuited to the post. The language about Henry used by the Yorkist rebels, even when Richard, Duke of York finally did claim the throne for himself, did not actually allude to Henry's mental troubles. There is no indication that he, any more than anyone else in charge,[342] thought it in any way disqualified him from the throne.

The reason for this would not have been acceptance of mental illness as inevitable and a matter of God, and as such not something that actually prevented Henry from performing his duties as king, and therefore, by mediaeval understanding, God's anointed. Instead, there was some sort of fear of fate or God involved in it, the knowledge that it had happened to Henry, as far as Richard and his adherents were concerned, without warning. Presumably, in case of something like it ever happening to Richard himself or his descendants, they did not wish for a precedent to be set, a chance to remove them from the throne on the same grounds as Richard had removed Henry VI.

The legitimate fear of actual mental illness might then have motivated Richard and his adherents to choose this course of action in attacking both Henry's ancestry and his actions. The choice was a miserable one, in some ways, but one that came as a matter of course to usurpation:

there needed to be an unassailable explanation that at the same time was not actually possible to replicate and be used against the person doing the usurping once he was on the throne. Therefore, generic accusations of allowing disorder were the safest bet, and this was what was used by Richard, Duke of York.[343]

Doubtlessly, his enemies would have wanted to use the same against him should they be able to remove him from power, but insanity was another level of problematic accusation to use. Richard could have used it with much more justification than anyone else in a similar position might have done. Not only did Henry actually suffer from a mental illness that occasionally made him unable not only to rule but even understand what was happening and give any opinion on what was happening, it was that very mental illness happening to Henry that first catapulted Richard, Duke of York into the position of ruler, and first drew many to him as a very effective ruler.

Even so, using this as a reason for Henry's removal from the throne was setting a precedent and less true accusations of mental illness could have been used against him and his descendants to attempt to usurp their throne, too. It would be a precedent that was uncomfortable at the very least, and the understanding of mental illness as has been explored in Chapter 2 shows that it could have extended far beyond that, too.

As has been discussed in Chapter 2, mental illness was often not regarded as too different from physical illness in many aspects, especially if it was a high-born man or woman struck down with it. There was a lot in the treatment and reception of Henry VI's mental illness that echoed the reception of a physical illness in kings, and in many ways, presumably it would have been treated the same way had he been in a coma after an accident or something similar.

Therefore, Richard, Duke of York using the mental illness Henry suffered from against him, as a reason as to why he was not suited to be king would not only create a precedent for him and his descendants, with even a rumour of mental illness (real or concocted) becoming dangerous to them and their hold on the throne, it could also have been otherwise problematic: even a mere physical illness could have presented a huge problem for them, with enemies claiming that it made them unable to properly hold onto the throne and fulfil their kingly tasks. As such, it was in Richard's interest to ignore the obvious accusation against Henry, or rather the obvious fact to use as to why he should not be king.

This also meant that he looked like a good man with a simple grievance of having had his inheritance stolen by Henry VI's grandfather, rather than someone with a grievance about Henry VI's ruling. Someone who saw Henry as his rightful king but refused to take him as he was, someone who thereby actively went against God's wishes, as would have been believed at the time, would have been harder to justify. That he did not choose that option helped him in his standing not only in England, of course, but also in other European countries, and as a matter of fact, even ensured the Pope sided with him.[344] Ignoring the most obvious and well-known fact was therefore not a gesture of kindness on his part, a gesture that showed that mental illnesses were not actually reviled, but simply a clever political manoeuvre.

Moreover, he must have been aware of the fact that while he and his adherents avoided the subject of Henry's mental illness, his supporters would not and would, in fact, mention it often enough for it to be seen as a factor in why Henry VI was not considered a rightful king. This, too, was nothing very new or something that was only limited to kings suffering from mental illnesses. On the contrary; then as now, rumours and even smear campaigns were rarely connected with the people in whose name they were run, even if they had given the orders for it. This could be anything from sexual slanders to accusations of not being the rightful king due to not being the son of their father, to mental illness. In fact, there is some evidence that Richard, Duke of York had run just such a smear campaign some years previously, against his political enemy and Henry VI's close advisor William, Duke of Suffolk, very successfully too.[345] It made William highly unpopular in all of England, causing violent hate against him that eventually saw him losing his life. All this was done, though, in such a way that there was no actual proof to tie Richard, Duke of York to it. As such, he must have been aware he could see Henry's mental illness used against him without ever having to do it himself.

This is what happened, whether Richard actually intended it to happen or not. Several of his modern-day defenders insist that it was not his intention and that the very fact he had spent years serving Henry faithfully without any due reward and had spent years attacking everyone around him but not the king himself showed he did not actually carry any ill-will towards Henry. This is perfectly possible, but of course sheer guesswork. It is definitely a fact that by 1460, when he claimed the throne in his own right, this was a clear declaration of war against Henry, and whether his motives were ill-will or not is irrelevant.

Even if he did not actually have any bad feelings towards the king, but felt pressured to take this course of action, this does not mean that he did not at the very least indicate his willingness to have whatever accusation there was used against Henry. It would only have been a logical political course of action. It is notable that even though those supporting the Yorkists did use Henry's mental illness against him, there was once more no actual vitriol used. Though there is plenty of vitriol towards other of his actions, his mental illness is once more treated very drily, for example in the Earl of Warwick's statement in 1460, saying that 'Our king is stupid and out of his mind: he does not rule but is ruled'.[346] Though hinting at Henry's mental illness, it does not actually spell it out, instead it just makes the point that he was not intelligent enough to avoid being manipulated. That he was manipulated was obviously the key point of Warwick's statement, rather than Henry's supposed 'stupidity'.

Though the language is insulting to modern ears, the fact he suffered from a mental illness is no attack on Henry himself, simply a statement as to his unsuitability as a king, which is a fair point. The statement is mostly true in itself, even if it somewhat exaggerates the effects of Henry's illness, in a stylistic choice very common of political condemnations of the time.

It is obvious that the circumstances were not the same for others suffering from the same afflictions that Henry did, or from any other mental illness. The assumption often appears to be that those of lesser standing were treated less well, but this is not necessarily the case. There were problems inherent in being a commoner suffering from a mental illness which did not concern nobility or royalty suffering in the same way, but the same is true vice versa as well. Henry VI's illness put him under the greatest possible scrutiny, it saw people he cared for disadvantaged and eventually, it was a deciding factor in his own downfall, for reasons that were not his fault.

Again, it could be argued that this was not too uncommon a consequence of mental illness and that Henry VI eventually ended up in prison as well. If one follows this argument, one has to also see that this was not directly due to his mental illness. Once Edward IV captured Henry VI after gaining the throne, he had little other choice but to treat him as any other usurper before him had treated the king he had usurped and have him imprisoned. The same had happened to Richard II and Edward II so any connection between Henry's mental illness and his imprisonment is at best implicit. It could be argued that had he not been mentally ill, the opportunity for Richard, Duke of York and his descendants to usurp his throne would never have arisen, but this is a rather tenuous claim considering England's history ever since Henry IV had usurped the throne. While Henry VI's mental illness did indeed offer a political opportunity to Richard, Duke of York, there is no way to say if he would not have found just such an opportunity had Henry VI become physically too ill to reign in 1453, rather than mentally. As such, while Henry's usurpation and eventual imprisonment followed directly from the circumstances surrounding his worst attack of mental illness, it cannot be said to have definitely caused them and that he suffered through this explicitly because of his mental illness. Moreover, there was a concerted effort made by Richard, Duke of York and Edward IV to explicitly not blame Henry's mental illness for anything they did, and to instead present Henry's actions when sane as the cause for their subsequent actions.

However, not all monarchs in this position were as lucky. The case of Juana La Loca was exactly the opposite. She was removed from power by her own father *because* she was supposedly so badly mentally ill that she could not rule, and she was imprisoned because her supposed mental illness allegedly meant she was unable to live on her own without being watched. Nor was Juana's imprisonment even in a mental hospital, where she could at least have received the correct care that she supposedly needed for her illness. Instead she was sent to prison.[347]

Again, the political reasons for this are obvious. Since Ferdinand's claim to rule Castile came from the very same woman as Juana's came — his wife and Juana's mother Isabella — he could not declare that she had no claim at all, the way Richard, Duke of York did with Henry VI. Moreover, he could not allow her to be at large, for the same reason as Henry VI was eventually not allowed to be at large. Since, unlike Henry VI, she was not actually officially usurped, there had to be another reason for her imprisonment. This has to be taken into account when comparing her case to Henry's, and trying to understand the English response to that of other countries — in this specific case, Spain's.

Not surprisingly, being imprisoned did not help Juana's condition, whatever this condition actually was. She was never freed again; after her father's death, her son took over as his regent, and Juana, despite being the queen regnant, never actually got to fulfil that role.[348]

There is a debate put forward by historians as to whether Juana had, by then, become so mentally ill that her son considered it unwise, if not downright impossible, to let her rule, or whether he simply continued with his grandfather's excuse,[349] deciding that he wanted to be regent and that his mother had to stay imprisoned for that to work. There is a suggestion that Juana did actually try to rule in her own name[350] but did not succeed, something which has been taken as evidence that she was as mentally ill as her father and later her son claimed.[351] This suggests that while their treatment of her was despicable, the claim of Juana's so-called madness it was based on was actually correct. None of Juana's actions or her failure to rule serve to confirm this though. The main problem, that she never properly tried to overcome, perhaps being aware of its utter impossibility, was that she was widely considered as mad after nearly one and a half decades of her father claiming just that. It seems that the fact that Juana was technically queen regnant and as such entitled to rule in her own right, without having to take the advice of her father and her son, was only mentioned if it served to spite either of them, and was never, at any point, used by someone willing to fight for her rights.

This is definitely interesting and is another contrast to Henry VI. He was known to have had attacks of mental illness, the worst of which rendered him unable not only to rule but actually react for over a year, but he still had nobles ready to fight for him and die for his right to be on the throne. The difference may be that Juana was a woman, and that mental illness in her was therefore treated differently than it was in a man, another subject that will be addressed below. The difference could also be that Juana had never ruled in her own right and that there would have been hesitancy to let someone rule who was claimed and widely believed to be mad. When she died at the age of 75, she was known as Juana the Mad, and this is the way she has been remembered down the centuries; even today it is the title of her Wikipedia article.

As mentioned previously, this complete amalgamation of the mental illness with the person suffering from it is something that also happened to Charles VI and Henry VI in history books, and in some ways, Juana's historiography fits in very well with theirs. However, for her, unlike for them, it happened in her lifetime. Not only was her mental illness used to strip her of her power and her regency, it was also used to strip her of her very personality, in the public eye as well as in the eyes of her own family.[363]

Some of the documents that show Ferdinand and Charles's thoughts about their daughter and mother still survive[364] and they very much indicate that they saw her as a nuisance, both politically and privately. None of the compassion extended even by strangers to Henry VI and, to a lesser extent, Charles VI was shown by them. At the very best, they ordered treatments for her that they may have actually considered would help, but without making any arrangements for her eventually getting better.[365] At worst, they actively stoked resentment and prejudice against her, using her mental illness as a weapon.[366] There is no indication of any sort of compassion, let alone love, in any of these documents, in which Juana is treated as if her mental illness makes her a lesser human.

There are two possible reasons for this, which need to be examined to have a more complete picture of the understanding and treatment of mental illness during the mediaeval and early modern times in Europe. One possibility is that, for all modern prejudices towards France and England during that time, there was a better understanding or a kinder disposition towards mentally ill people in those countries at the time. The other possibility is one that is often alluded to in discussions about Juana and her mental illness: that the difference was not a cultural one but simply one of gender. Juana was a woman and Henry VI and Charles VI men, and as such afforded more compassion.

This is an idea that has become especially widespread in recent decades and has even led to some rather polemic statements, such as by Salvatore Poeta[367] who stated that there was a general distaste for women inheriting thrones in the first place at the time and men worked to prevent that. He also argued that women who did in fact become heir to a throne could be exploited by men wishing to have some of their powers.

For a proper discussion of the subject though, no such claims and statements can be simply taken as fact but need to be examined to see if they fit with the available evidence. The very first bit of this claim, for one, does not and seems to be judged mostly on Victorian ideas of English inheritance laws, rather than any actual mediaeval laws and ideas, much less mediaeval Spanish ideas. In England at that time, there was indeed only one case of a woman inheriting the throne, a case that had not ended well. In France, they had Salic law in place, which meant that women were prohibited from inheriting the throne at all. None of this had ever happened in Spain. In fact, Juana's mother, Isabella of Castile, was both very powerful and very well respected, with there being no indication that anyone thought she was a lesser ruler because she was a woman, or that it would have been better had a man inherited instead of her.

Moreover, Isabella herself was rather involved in sowing the seeds of her daughter Juana being considered mad, and quite possibly, even in actually causing her mental illness, at least as much as Ferdinand himself. This will be examined in more detail in Chapter 4, but it is well known that Isabella very much opposed her daughter's stand on a number of things, deeply disagreed with her religiously and was known to consider Juana's religious opinions 'madness' and to refer to them as such.[368] Therefore, the opposition to Juana as a regent and the reaction to her so-called madness were not solely inspired by misogyny, a desire to discredit any woman with a strong claim to be ruler or anything of the sort. If anything, it was religiously motivated at first.

However, the second part of Poeta's statement is more immediately correct. While a woman marrying a king regnant only became a queen consort, with no right to actually rule the country, a man marrying a queen regnant became a king and effectively her co-ruler. This of course put queen regnants at a distinct disadvantage to king regnants and in many ways was an invitation for greedy noblemen to try and become a king, while relying on the fact that male rulers were more widespread to effectively gain more power than their wives. This was not always the case, as could be seen from the union of Juana's parents, as Isabella of Castile knew how to defend her own rights. It was, however, the first reason for the dispute between Juana's husband Philip the Handsome and her father Ferdinand, as both of these men considered he should be her co-ruler, something that would not have happened had she been a man and considered to be perfectly able to rule alone. While Isabella of Castile had stressed her own right to rule alone, she had never actually done so and as such, it would be up to whichever man won the power struggle to rule alongside Juana.[369]

That Juana was not even asked who she preferred as her co-ruler is rather telling as to how dismissively she was treated, though it is hard to say if this was due to misogyny or her mental illness, or a mixture thereof. By comparison, once their mental illness had manifested, there were times when neither Henry VI nor Charles VI were in the position to make decisions for themselves and the country they ruled, and as such, were actually in the same position as Juana. However, in their cases the decisions made to safeguard their rule were not as long-lasting and not quite as important as the decision made against Juana and her province of Castile she was meant to rule. Since it was only because she was a woman that it was even considered she needed any co-regent at all. And even if the motives of her husband and father were solely concerned with her mental illness and they legitimately thought they were acting in her best interests by seeing to it she had one of them as her co-regent, the very nature of the problem they were discussing was rooted in misogyny.

However, for all the comparative kindness experienced by other royals who suffered from mental health problems in the Middle Ages, it would perhaps be more accurate to say that most of Juana's problems stemmed from her mental illness, rather from her being female, and prejudices connected with perceptions of women being rulers. It could be comparatively unproblematic: her mother ruled in her own name with great success. If a woman was not desired as ruler, purely because of her sex, there was also a precedent for that. The most famous example for this in England is the case of Empress Matilda, who in the twelfth century was usurped by her cousin King Stephen, with the actual reasoning that a man was a better ruler than a woman, and therefore the nephew of a deceased king was his natural heir over his daughter. This was accepted by some, but by no means by everyone

Part of the problem for Juana was that there was no obvious male candidate to take over the job, but Ferdinand and Philip could have tried saying that although they ruled by right of her, she was not actually suited to ruling herself due to being a woman. That this was not tried and never once was her mental illness connected to the strain of being the heiress to two monarchs, and later being an actual monarch herself, certainly shows that, despite the example of Empress Matilda, there was no existing prejudice against women monarchs strong enough to tap into, to use to exclude her from the throne on this alone.[370]

Even so, the connection between how Juana's mental illness was treated in comparison to the male Henry VI and Charles VI and their respective genders should not be ignored completely. After all, it has often been suggested that Juana's mental illness was but a pretext to see her excluded from the throne of Castile, explicitly because she was a woman and her father Ferdinand did not want to have a woman on the throne of Castile.[371]

This argument is, however, somewhat spurious. The only claim Ferdinand himself had to the throne of Castile was through his wife, and he was very happy for her to rule Castile during her lifetime. While Isabella was a forceful and strong woman, who is unlikely to have reacted well had her husband ever tried ruling in her name or even tried to usurp some of her powers, there is no evidence he ever even tried.[372] Therefore, it could be that had Juana's brother Juan, who died as a teenager, been in her exact position, that Ferdinand would have reacted exactly the same as he did for Juana. It is, however, likely that while he himself simply wanted to not give up the power of being ruler over Castile as well as Aragon, that he knew that such behaviour would be more accepted towards his daughter than towards a son.

The other possibility is that there was more prejudice against mental illness in Spain during mediaeval and early modern times than there was in France or England and that this informed both Ferdinand and indeed Isabella's reaction towards their daughter, It would also explain the more widespread acceptance of terrible treatment towards Juana because of her illness than there would have been for such treatment of Charles VI or Henry VI in France or England respectively.

The opposite is often claimed to have happened, with Spain in many cases being presented as a sort of respite of culture and knowledge as opposed to the terrible and dank Middle Ages in the rest of Europe, thanks to the conquest by the Moors some centuries before. However, while it is still a sadly widespread idea, this has already been thoroughly debunked by many historians over the last century. It is true that due to the conquest, Spain and its culture were changed and new ideas were accepted. However, the idea that it was the Moorish conquerors who taught Europeans to wash, or to make use of medicines, as well as assorted other skills, stems from a Victorian misreading about the European Middle Ages. It is factually wrong.[373]

The same can be said about 'Moorish' and Spanish medicine. Since it was a whole other culture, there were different ideas which circulated, for both physical and mental illnesses. However, that these cures, treatments and ideas were always better and more enlightened is not something that is supported by the evidence at all. As such, it is perfectly possible that there was a different and more hostile attitude towards people suffering from mental illness in Spain than there was in France or in England at the time.[374]

Another claim that is often made is that by Isabella and Ferdinand's counter-conquest, a lot of previously enlightened ideas were instantly lost. This is harder to disprove, since it would mean proving a negative, but it is still rather a spurious claim. There can be no doubt that Isabella and Ferdinand were very cruel, especially in their religious ideals, which led to some of the worst excesses of late mediaeval Christianity and moreover saw the horrible move of the expulsion of all Jewish people from their realms. Doubtlessly, this lost Spain a lot of interesting and positive influences on cultures and ideas, including medical developments. However, the idea of there being a sudden loss of knowledge, and an immediate cultural decline, which influenced any and all parts of life, is simply not supported by any of the existing evidence.

Even if there was a stark and strong fear of going against what Isabella and Ferdinand ordered, particularly religiously, and an understandable hesitation to say or do anything that might upset them, particularly by holding unorthodox beliefs, this would not immediately have changed the existing cultural norms. While nothing would have been said to openly contradict the king and queen, this does not mean there would immediately have been a change from a belief set held for several hundred years. The idea that due to the conquest of Iberia, Spain had held enlightened and progressive beliefs, in stark contrast to the rest of Europe from the eighth century onwards, only to immediately plunge back into the supposed Dark Ages upon the strictly, even for the time fundamentally, religious Ferdinand and Isabella's reconquest, would require everyone to change their beliefs practically overnight, an absolute impossibility. Therefore, for Ferdinand to choose his daughter's mental illness to discredit her in the public mind, there must have been a stigma to mental illness that did not exist to this extent elsewhere in Europe at the time, and this must have been a stigma that had been some while in the making, although the sources are scarce.

Of course, there is a way that Ferdinand and Isabella did change the definition of mental illness, a way that also included how they saw their own daughter Juana. This was to do with their perception of Christian doctrine and belief, which will be discussed below. However, as will also be seen, this sort of belief — the idea that a Christian belief system that was in any way different to their own very strict one, let alone any other religion — constituted mental illness, was very much one that was imposed by them, not one that was, so to speak, grown organically by their people.

As to the actual truth or lack thereof of Spain being less tolerant and more prejudiced towards mentally ill people, there is very little to say, as almost all trials in Juana's lifetime were somehow connected with religion.[375] As such it is hard to find any independent information on the perception of mental illness and its cures and treatments.

Even so, it is interesting to note that contemporary sources show that both Henry VI and Charles VI were treated far better. This might be a cultural difference, but there was another factor for Juana that did not happen for either of them: Juana was not yet ruler when her mental illness,[376] whatever it actually was, took hold and as such it was far easier to stop her from gaining power that she may very well have been considered unfit for. Once, however, a monarch was ruler and had been crowned, it was much harder to take this rule away. Since a coronation involved being anointed by God, this meant, by the belief system of the fifteenth and sixteenth centuries, that God Himself had chosen and approved of the person as ruler. To consider someone unsuited for it was one thing before it happened, but after it had happened, it became much more difficult. Juana was not crowned, and so it was easier to treat her as not being able to rule, and also to actually speak against her in general. This might also be part of why Juana felt the full force of prejudice against mental illness, while Henry and Charles did not, rather than any cultural differences.

However, this presupposes that other people suffering from mental illnesses, who were not royalty, were all treated at least as badly as Juana, if not worse. There is little evidence for or against that in Spain, but there is enough evidence to say that this was most definitely not the case in France or England.

One such case that has been addressed above is that of George Neville, Lord Latimer, who became mentally ill during adulthood at one point and became a ward of his brother. Contemporarily, this was said to be due to 'the love' his brother had for him. However, despite this, the idea that he was punished by no longer being allowed to keep his lands for himself is one that is still rather widespread, which is an interesting idea, but fails to take into account the very strong possibility that George actually did suffer from a mental illness, which is definitely suggested by the fact that his family never protested against him being dispossessed by reason of his supposed 'idiocy'. Unless everyone, including his own wife and son, who were themselves disadvantaged by this dispossession, colluded to strip George of his possessions for showing the tiniest sign of a mental illness, it can be said with reasonable certainty that he actually did suffer from a severe form of mental illness, rendering him unable to cope with the demands of managing his own lands and possessions.

With this being the case, George's brother being his guardian and taking over the management of his estates for him, working in his best interest, is not something that is a punishment, or even unusual. Even today, a guardian is appointed in the case of someone becoming mentally too unwell to take care of their own business and their own possessions. The idea of something similar happening in the Middle Ages being seen as a punishment, rather than a necessity, indicates more the prejudices with which modern historians regard the Middle Ages and judge every action with the worst possible assumptions. Such assumptions often ignore similar actions which still exist today and says more about the kind of prejudices that are prevalent today with regards to the Middle Ages, than shining any light on mediaeval actions surrounding mental illnesses and the people suffering from them. As a matter of fact, George Neville, Lord Latimer's case serves rather well to showcase that our ways of dealing with adults afflicted with mental illness that renders them unable to function in the real world, does not differ too much from that of our mediaeval forebears. It is just as likely that even today a rich person who finds themselves suffering from a mental illness and unable to take care of their own vast possessions might be given, together with their lands, into the care of a relative.

George's is just one example, discussed in more detail in Chapter 2, but his story illustrates well that one didn't have to have had a coronation or be 'chosen by God' to inform people's behaviour towards those with a mental illness.

3.1. Legal ramifications of mental illness

Juana's case suggests that there was a lot to be gained from having a relative declared insane, and that it was comparatively easy to do so, even to a monarch. However, Juana was a special case. It does not seem that it was commonly very easy, though it changed from case to case. There may indeed have been cases in which the decision to declare someone legally insane was made by the king on the insistence of relatives, with little to no cause to do so at all.

Mostly, however, it seems that there was a set of rules in place, which were required to be followed to declare someone mentally ill, and, for the purposes of those doing so, not only mentally ill but actually unable to control their possessions, be able to make life decisions and otherwise function like a normal adult in everyday life.[377] As has been seen above, there had to be quite a case to be able be granted someone's possessions, and in that case, it usually went to someone who was sympathetic to the mentally ill person, someone who could be trusted to take good care of them and the stricken person themself. There could have been cases in which someone acted as if they wanted to manage someone's possessions in the best possible way and then used it for their own gain, but on the whole, it seems as if such cases were rare.

The most examples we have for someone being declared insane in late mediaeval England refer to noblemen and noblewomen, whose lives were far more recorded than those of commoners. Not only that, but since nearly all noble families were significantly richer than any and all commoner families, one of their own being declared insane would also have far more fiscal consequences.

Consequently, if someone did want their relative declared insane, a member of the nobility would have had far more to gain from it than a commoner. However, most noblemen also had a strong system of supporters and men and women working for them, so it would have been rather difficult to have someone declared insane without, at the very least, someone protesting, and, more likely than not, things erupting into actual violence.[378] Not only might their household and dependents have protested, but also the nobleman or noblewoman in question herself, so that it would be all but impossible to do it without there being at least some underlying cause, a hint of the person in question actually suffering from mental illness.

Finally, though mental illness was not actually as badly stigmatised as is often claimed, as can be seen especially in the cases of William, Viscount Beaumont and George, Lord Latimer, it was still not something many would have voluntarily associated with. Mental illness as well as physical disability were reasons to reject an arranged marriage,[379] and though being related to someone who was mentally ill was not, there would still have been the danger of it 'rubbing off' on the reputation of the nobleman in question, lessening the chances for marriage of him- or herself and his or her children.

It would have to go further than that, however far 'that' was, for someone to be actually declared insane because of any sort of unusual behaviour. What exactly such behaviour was is hard if not downright impossible to say. There is no hint at all towards what it was that saw George Neville, Lord Latimer, so labelled and why the king considered him unable to take care of his own lands and possessions. Due to the lack of protest not only from him but also from his own relatives, who would have had every reason to protest at this had they considered it unjust, it stands to reason that they all agreed on him being mentally too unwell to be trusted with business. Even so, he was considered well enough to take care of himself. If ever this changed, it was at least never officially put to parliament. This means that his behaviour must have been strange enough to be considered obvious 'idiocy', yet not bad enough to justify stripping him of his own autonomy.

Since there is an absolute lack of records about George Neville's behaviour that caused him to be declared mentally ill, no judgement or comparison can be made to see any difference between his behaviour and that of contemporaries who were also declared mentally unwell.

Thankfully, there is somewhat more evidence for us to know why William Beaumont, Viscount Beaumont, was declared insane. His behaviour, that saw his lands and possessions handed over to his friend John de Vere, Earl of Oxford, appears to have been that he spent large amounts of money and, there is an indication that not only that, but that he gave away large chunks of his lands as well, to such an extent that it was considered harmful behaviour both for himself and any heirs he might have.

This sounds fairly sensible to modern ears, but it does beg the question just how extreme this was, or where the difference was to other nobles spending a lot of money and selling parts of their lands. It was common for noblemen in the fifteenth and sixteenth centuries, and in fact in the years before and afterwards as well, to have massive debts. A typical example for this is Elizabeth of York, Queen Consort of Henry VII, whose debts are legendary,[380] yet who was never considered to be mentally unwell because of it, or even so much as unusual for continuing to spend large amounts of money she obviously did not have. Even if the reasoning behind it was that the person in question had to realise what he or she was doing, that overspending was not a sign of madness and mental illness as long as it was clear that the person was fully aware of their incurring debts, not everyone seems to have been considered mad for not fulfilling these criteria. William Beaumont's brother-in-law, John Lovell, Baron Lovell, ran up such extreme debts that he had to sell two of his manors in 1462, due to owing two men more than £1000, and it did not even make a dent in his debts.[381] Despite this, despite the fact that these debts seemed to come from uncontrolled behaviours — and despite, notably, John Lovell, Baron Lovell being a widely despised man, whom many would doubtlessly have liked to see stripped of his lands and possessions — he was never at all considered in any way mad, and no one ever commented on his mental health.

Obviously, William Beaumont's behaviour must have been more extreme than that, though just how that is possible is hard to fathom. Perhaps it was not just extreme spending, but also the whys and wherefores of that spending that was used to judge whether the person doing the spending was simply a bad businessman who did not care about debts, or if they were actually mentally ill. How this was done is sadly unknown to us, but a possibility is suggested to us by the very fact that in the two cases we know most about, that of William Beaumont and that of George Latimer, the lands and possessions were taken by someone quite close to them. It is therefore possible that these men, John de Vere Earl of Oxford and Richard Neville Earl of Salisbury, could judge their behaviour best and noticed a change in them, a change so extreme it could not be natural and was in flagrant contrast to all their previous behaviour. This is however only speculation and cannot be used as actual evidence for how such things were judged.

William Beaumont's case is of special interest, because as mentioned above, eight years after he was considered too mentally unwell to take care of his lands, he was also declared too mentally unwell to take care of himself. What behaviour led to this is sadly also sheer guesswork, but obviously, it must have been worse, or at the very least extreme enough for this to have become notable. With him being unable to overspend, this could not have been caused by any sort of mismanagement of money and must have referred to personal behaviour. In fact, it was especially stressed that his behaviour, if not checked, would embarrass not only him but also the king, since William was a member of the nobility.

Again, this must have been behaviour widely judged to be outside of the norm. Since there was a wide array of behaviour considered somewhat mad by modern standards but normal by the standards of the fifteenth and sixteenth centuries, once more we can only judge that it must have been extreme and against all the then accepted norms. This is all the more so because there was actually no way that anyone, neither the king nor John de Vere, who had custody of William's possessions, profited from it. On the contrary, leaving William to his own devices and seeing only to it that he had enough money to support himself, would have doubtlessly profited John de Vere much more than having his custody, having to take care of him and pay for his upkeep. Therefore, his behaviour must have indeed actually been rather mad, whatever this meant by the standards of the late fifteenth century. Presumably, this means that what was said in the grant giving John de Vere, Earl of Oxford, custody of his friend William Beaumont, was at least roughly correct.

Just what this means is pure guesswork, but the very fact that his behaviour was considered embarrassing to the king if it continued shows that it must have not only been fairly extreme,[382] but almost certainly gone against the accepted standards of society. Notably, since this echoes the language used for Juana of Castile somewhat, it could be that this 'madness' was in some way connected to religion, that William went against the accepted belief sets of Christianity that all nobles were expected to hold. While there are cases in which it was implicitly accepted that noblemen and noblewomen in the Middle Ages did not quite share these beliefs, or expressed doubts, and while this belief set was nowhere near as static as is often believed, it was still expected that there should be no blatant transgression against the teachings of the Church.

As such, we can assume that unless we explicitly know otherwise, those who were declared to be unable to take care of themselves or their lands, whose land and sometimes wardship were handed to close relatives or friends, did in fact suffer from a mental illness and that caring for them in a kind way was a priority to their relatives as well as, in many cases, also the king.

If someone were said to be slightly simple, then often this was used as a reason as to why they could not inherit. Therefore, mental illness could be used as an accusation, something to discredit someone and disadvantage them. There are some such cases recorded, though it does not seem as if they were always very successful.[383] Though in many cases, it was an accusation that would stick, in rumours if nothing else, more often than not, the accusations did not achieve what they intended, and did not cause the person to be considered unable to do business, and therefore assume an inheritance.

The accusation of so-called 'insanity' was not the only one, of course, used against a rival in inheritance cases or in other ways. It was only one in a stable of such excuses and accusations, which also included false paternity, accusations of crimes, and simple claims of wrong birth order. Mental illness was, in fact, much more rarely used than any of those, but when it was used, it was generally solved in the same ways as other such cases: with witnesses being brought to disprove the argument.[384]

Inheritance disputes in particular were hardly unusual in mediaeval England and also in mediaeval France, and while there were rare cases in which it was solved by two brothers, two sisters or two couples agreeing privately, more often than not these did end up in court, where all litigants tried to prove that their opponent did not have a right. Often, this was done by disputing a will, but not infrequently, there was also an attempt to smear the opponent or prove by personal tales that he or she was not entitled to their share of the inheritance.[385]

Claims of insanity was one of these tales,[386] and as with claims of the defendant not being the deceased's real son or daughter, or that they were, in fact, later in the birth order than claimed and therefore not entitled to the inheritance share they received, it was one that relied on witnesses which were handpicked by the defendant or the claimant, to prove their case. Such witnesses were not always reliable, and in many cases there is evidence of bribery to get these witnesses to say what was required.

In the face of this, it is interesting that insanity was an accusation far less often brought than the other claims, and also one of the least likely to succeed, though the former could result from the latter. What we learn from this is that it was considered harder to prove someone was mentally ill, or at least mentally ill to such an extent as to bar them from inheriting something, than it was to prove or convince a judge that someone was, in fact, the result of an affair, a cuckoo child, or younger than originally claimed.

This suggests that mental illness, while sometimes used as slander, was not particularly effective as such compared to other accusations.

It also means that, contrary to what is often claimed, there is actually no evidence whatsoever of the mere accusation of mental health issues being enough to destroy someone's reputation or of mentally ill people being hated so much that it was the ultimate accusation.

3.2. Accusations of insanity and weird behaviour

Whether the same held true for most commoners declared mentally unfit to take care of themselves and their possessions is far harder to know, of course. The same principles would at least theoretically have applied to them: that there was a fiscal advantage for any relative of a person declared insane, but also that there was a social disadvantage in being closely related to someone who would have been called 'a lunatic' at the time. Naturally, there is not much evidence about individual cases. While some names and the mental illness they were diagnosed with survive, there is nothing by way of information as to their possessions, their family and similar details which could make even a rudimentary guess as to the reason for their being declared so possible. All we can do, therefore, is go by what information there is for those sections of the population which were recorded, and make assumptions from those details, while keeping in mind it may not actually be correct for all sections of the population.

As a matter of fact, there is something of a suggestion that rather than people being declared mentally ill at a whim, and then promptly ostracised for good, that the opposite was the case and that behaviour patterns that are seen as indicative of mental illness today were not seen as that during the Middle Ages and early modern period. There are several people who are now often assumed to have suffered from some sort of mental illness, whose behaviour seems to indicate it for modern-day researchers, but who were not considered mentally ill at the time, and their behaviour not judged as such at all.

As has been seen above, this even counts for people who manifested symptoms we know today are a sign of a mental illness, such as hearing voices. This was, however, seen as somewhat unusual, even if it was explained in a distinctly different way to today, and a religious explanation was offered instead of a medical one. Other unusual behaviour, which could be indicative of a mental illness, was often simply accepted as normal and expected, even if it were occasionally judged. A perfect example for this is George, Duke of Clarence, younger brother of Edward IV and older brother of Richard III. It is all but accepted in modern-day biographies of him and his brothers that he was not entirely mentally healthy. This is treated with varying degrees of sympathy from the author Charles Ross saying his behaviour was 'foolish' and using 'mad'[387] as a slur, to author John Ashdown-Hill stressing the possibility of his possible mental health problems as an excuse for his behaviour.[388] Most authors fall between these two extremes.

It is possible that the modern-day tendency to diagnose a man who was not contemporarily noted to even have a hint of mental illness is simply influenced by the knowledge of what George actually went through in his life, which today would almost certainly mean he would have to go to therapy to make sure he properly got to deal with it all.

The list of potentially traumatic events George went through is long. His father and brother were killed when he was 11 years old. Following this, he was sent into exile with his 8-year-old brother, because their mother feared that they, too, might be targets. During his teenage years, he was treated with little interest, if not downright contempt by his brother Edward IV, which caused George to betray him to side with his father-in-law several years later. He found his father-in-law disappointed his expectations as well and his wife lost a child due to actions he might have blamed on said father-in-law. So, George went against him again to side with his brother. Following this, he spent some time arguing with his younger brother about his and his wife's rights to several of their possessions, and finally lost his wife and his baby in short succession. Given all this, it would not be surprising if George actually did suffer from a form of mental illness, although possibly nothing more than slight paranoia or PTSD. However, though it is often treated as that today, it is hardly a given. George's situation was not as unique as it sounds and many of his contemporaries went through similarly horrible experiences, even as children, without being considered mentally ill either at the time or today, and without their behaviour ever suggesting anything of the like. George's own brother Richard, his sister Margaret and his brother-in-law John, Duke of Suffolk, are prime examples of that.

Naturally, that does not mean that George did not actually suffer from a mental illness. We know today, as people knew during the late mediaeval period, that people react differently to stress and that situations that were easily dealt with by many or even most could prove too much for others. It is perfectly conceivable that this was the case for George also; that he found it harder to cope with what he had gone through than other members of his family and that it triggered a mental illness. It is, however, also possible that he simply was not mentally ill and that his somewhat erratic behaviour was simply his normal modus operandi, as seemed to be thought during his own lifetime.

That his behaviour was somewhat erratic and certainly showed a paranoid streak, especially in the last years of his life, is hard to deny. Centuries worth of propaganda have made working out what his behaviour was actually like difficult, but some of it is recorded in the parliamentary rolls:

> To the most wise and discreet commons assembled in this present parliament; Roger Twynyho, cousin and heir of Ankarette, widow of William Twynyho of Cayford in the county of Somerset, esquire, that is to say son of John, son of the said William and Ankarette, lamentably complains and shows in the most piteous and humble way to your great wisdoms, [*col. b*] that where the said Ankarette on Saturday 12 April in the seventeenth year of the reign of our present most dread sovereign lord the king [1477] was in her manor at Cayford aforesaid, in God's peace and that of our said sovereign lord, one Richard Hyde, late of Warwick in the county of Warwick, gentleman, and Roger Strugge, late of Beckhampton in the county of Somerset, fuller, accompanied by various riotous and mis-ruled persons, equipped and assembled in manner of war and insurrection, numbering eighty persons and more, at the command of George, duke of Clarence, intending by his craftily plotted schemings, groundless and baseless, contrary to all right, truth and conscience, the complete destruction and death of the said Ankarette, came to Cayford aforesaid at about two o'clock in the afternoon on the abovesaid day and in the said year; and then and there, with great fury and frenzy, broke into and entered the said Ankarette's house by force against the king's peace, and then and there took and imprisoned the same Ankarette, who was of good name and reputation,

without a writ, warrant or any other lawful authority; and they immediately carried and conveyed the said Ankarette, as a prisoner, from there the same day with great violence to the city of Bath in the same county without stopping, not allowing her to tarry in her own house to take some rest, or any of her servants to accompany her, and under similar duress carried and conveyed her from Bath aforesaid on the following Sunday to the town of Cirencester in the county of Gloucester, and from there conveyed her in the same way to the town of Warwick in the county of Warwick, and brought her there on the following Monday at about eight o'clock in the evening; which town of Warwick is seventy miles from the said manor of Cayford. And the said riotous persons, at the command of the said duke, immediately then [and] there took from the said Ankarette all such jewels, money, goods and chattels as she had there; and also then and there, on behalf of the said duke, as though he had used a king's power, commanded and firmly charged Thomas Delalynde, esquire, and Edith, his wife, the said Ankarette's daughter, and their other servants who had followed the said Ankarette in the hope of attending her, to take themselves away from the said town of Warwick, upon pain of death, and to lodge at Stratford upon Avon that night, which is six miles from there; on the strength of which command, and for fear of death, the said Thomas Delalynde and Edith, his wife, and their said other servants then departed from there without delay or tarrying, not being allowed to speak with the said Ankarette, and so they left her alone; and the said duke wrongfully kept the same Ankarette in such prison and duress there until the hour of six in the morning on Tuesday the following day, that is to say, the Tuesday next after the close of Easter [15 April]; and then with the same force and violence caused the said Ankarette to be brought to the Guildhall at Warwick aforesaid before some of the king's justices of the peace for the said county of Warwick, then sitting there in the king's general sessions of the peace in the same county; and then and there the said duke, to accomplish his said craftily plotted schemings, untruly and wickedly, contrary to all truth and conscience, brought pressure to bear so that she was indicted by the name of Ankarette Twynneowe, late of Warwick in the county of Warwick, widow, on the grounds that the said Ankarette, the former servant of George, duke of Clarence, and Isabel, his wife, [*memb. 11*] maliciously and damnably intending the destruction and death of the said Isabel at Warwick aforesaid, on 10 [*p. vi–174*][*col. a*] October in the sixteenth year of the reign of our said sovereign lord [1476] falsely, traitorously and feloniously gave the said Isabel a venomous drink of ale mixed with poison to drink, to poison and kill the said Isabel; of which drink the said Isabel sickened from the said 10 October until the Sunday next before the following Christmas [22 December]; on which Sunday she then and there died; and so the said Ankarette falsely, traitorously and feloniously killed the same Isabel there on the said Sunday. And immediately, on the same day, the said justices arraigned and made the said Ankarette answer to this; whereupon she pleaded that she was not guilty, whereupon by process made by the said justices the same day, a jury appeared and found the said Ankarette guilty of the matter contained in the said indictment; and thereupon it was decided and judged by the said justices that the said Ankarette should be led from the bar there to the king's gaol at Warwick aforesaid, and from that gaol she should be drawn through the centre of the said town of Warwick to the gallows at Myton, and be hanged on the said gallows until she was dead; and they commanded the sheriff of the said county then present to execute the judgment; and so he did: which indictment, trial and judgment were had, done and given within three hours on the said Tuesday, the same justices continuously sitting in the same sessions there without any adjournment of the said sessions during that time; a copy of all that record is attached to this. Which jurors, for fear and dread of great threats, and fearful of losing their lives and goods, reached the said verdict against their own wishes, truth and conscience; in proof of which various members of the same jury, after the said judgment had been given, came conscience-striken to the said Ankarette, knowing they had given an untrue verdict in that case, [and] humbly and piteously asked forgiveness for this from the said Ankarette.

The accusation brought by the king against the Duke of Clarence:

The king is mindful of the many conspiracies against him which he has repressed in the past, and although many of the rebels and traitors have been punished as an example to others yet, as a merciful prince, he spared not only the rank and file but also some of the movers and stirrers of such treasons. Notwithstanding, a conspiracy against him, the queen, their son and heir and a great part of the nobility of the land has recently come to his knowledge, which treason is more heinous and unnatural than any previous one because it originates from the king's brother the duke of Clarence, whom the king had always loved and generously rewarded. In spite of this, the duke grievously offended the king in the past, procuring his exile from the realm and labouring parliament to exclude him and his heirs from the crown. All of which the king forgave, but the duke continued to conspire against him, intending his destruction by both internal and external forces. He sought to turn his subjects against him by saying that Thomas Burdet was falsely put to death and that the king resorted to necromancy. He also said that the king was a bastard, not fit to reign, and made men take oaths of allegiance to him without excepting their loyalty to the king. He accused the king of taking his livelihood from him, and intending his destruction. He secured an exemplification under the great seal of an agreement made between him and Queen Margaret promising him the crown if Henry VI's line failed. He planned to send his son and heir abroad to win support, bringing a false child to Warwick castle in his place. He planned to raise war against the king within England and made men promise to be ready at an hour's notice. The duke has thus shown himself incorrigible and to pardon him would threaten the common weal, which the king is bound to maintain.

By the advice and assent of the lords and commons the king ordains that the duke be convicted of high treason and forfeit his estate as duke and all the lands he holds by the king's grant.

Answer: le roy le voet

Obviously, it is both possible that George simply decided to make as much trouble as he could for his brother the king, or that some of his behaviour was based on actual fears: for example, that Ankarette Twynyho actually had acted against him and poisoned his wife. But even so, his behaviour was still at the very least unusual. In both cases, the question as to why would have to be asked. The idea that Ankarette Twynyho actually did what George accused her of has been discussed in other books, with most coming to the conclusion that it is unlikely, and all pointing out that even if she did, George reacted rather strangely to it by not referring the matter to his brother the king, to go through the king's courts.[390] This would have been the usual course of action and George's failure to follow it already shows a tendency to mistrust the king. Though of course in the case of Ankarette actually being guilty, such fears would have been justified and his behaviour could hardly have been attributed to any sort of mental illness, or even behaviour that could indicate the danger of him becoming mentally ill.

However, if she were not guilty, as most historians think, his behaviour could definitely suggest that he was becoming clinically paranoid, if not outright suffering from this illness already. It has never been suggested that George simply wished to kill people for the sake of it or that he suffered from sociopathy and his behaviour certainly suggests nothing of the like.[391] This means that he, with absolutely no evidence that has survived until today, and according to all sources no evidence that anyone saw at the time, considered an elderly woman and a young man to be guilty of a crime that there is no evidence ever even happened. In modern terms, that is definitely not the sign of a healthy mind. It could, of course, be simply a sign that someone was playing him — there are plenty of examples, even from George's own lifetime — of men and women doing irrational things because they were manipulated into it for political gain.

This could be the case but would not explain his otherwise rather strange behaviour after the execution of Ankarette Twynyho and Sir Roger Tocotes, behaviour that was not only paranoid but downright self-destructive. Though some of George's actions, which have traditionally been considered as rather mad, such as his offering marriage to Mary, Duchess of Burgundy,[392] are perfectly sane and explicable by the standard of fifteenth-century politics, most of George's behaviour was not. For example, even if he was absolutely convinced of what he was doing and that his brother Edward IV was actually trying to demote and kill him, it does not seem like a very sensible course of action to openly act against Edward, contradict him at every turn possible and thereby give him more ammunition to act against him. In such a case, simply waiting Edward out and, if he needed to, quietly enact countermeasures would have made more sense.

One blatant example is that George became convinced that his brother Edward IV was trying to poison him, to the point of him even thinking Edward would do it openly at court. This would not have been far-fetched, considering the rough nature of fifteenth-century politics. There were a number of deaths in the fifteenth century attributed to supposed poison, though rarely was the king openly blamed. However, even blaming the king meant that George was committing treason, and as such giving his brother more reason to harm him than just quietly avoiding eating at court or using what was thought to be a unicorn horn, as an antidote.

George, instead, chose to make a huge production out of putting the powdered unicorn horn — which, as a matter of historical interest, was probably a narwhal tusk — in his drink while at court, making it plainly obvious that he considered Edward, and especially his wife, Queen Elizabeth Woodville, to be trying to kill him.[393]

There was another, rather ill-considered action which George, under any normal circumstances, must have known gave his brother a far cleaner chance to kill him rather than doing it secretly: he started insisting on his own claim to the throne, stressing that he was a prince and, it seems from his attainder, even insisting that the king's oldest son had no claim to the throne.

Due to what happened later, with Edward V actually being disinherited for reasons which are still debated and on the veracity of which historians still cannot agree, it has often been claimed that George was actually right about this. Even so, saying something that was so doubtlessly treason, regardless of its truth or lack thereof, was not a very clever move for someone who was afraid that his brother was seeking ways to kill him.

It has often been speculated that it was his wife's death that triggered a mental illness in him.[394] In fact, given what he had gone through in his life, this would hardly be unusual and the very fact that the Duchess of Clarence, Isabel Neville, died rather unexpectedly could have caused George to question the reason for her death. George's reaction to it would be unusual. While rumours and even claims of murder were only normal, and even kings were commonly implicated in them, actively assuming the king's authority to do what essentially amounted to a vigilante killing was a surefire way to self-destruction.

That this was caused by a mental illness seems obvious to everyone looking at his behaviour with twenty-first-century knowledge of mental health and mental health issues. It was behaviour that not only did not fit with George's previous behaviour in the first twenty-seven years of his life, but it also suggests that he was a stupid man, which he was definitely not.

In fact, despite the many claims of mental illness causing George's behaviour, there is still a lot of assumption that he was in fact not an intelligent man,[395] that seeks to square behaviour claimed to have been done while George suffered under a mental illness with his behaviour of the many years before and make it fit. This is faulty and suggests a connection between mental illness and stupidity that is problematic and not supported by any research.

The fact that all of George's actions, including those in his youth and the early part of his brother Edward IV's second reign, are seen through the lens of his supposed mental illness,[396] though behaviour that could be seen as connected to such a mental illness first manifested after 1475, is even more problematic than in Henry VI's case. For Henry VI, it also reveals a shocking prejudice in modern works against those suffering from mental illness, but in George's case, it presupposes not only that the modern reading is correct and that he did indeed suffer from clinical paranoia or some other sort of certifiable mental illness, but uses his previous actions to support this theory, while at the same time explaining these previous actions by this supposed mental illness. George's mental health, and problems with mental health, are therefore looked at with circular logic, that does not lead anywhere and shine any light on George's mental state.

In fact, neither by modern nor contemporary standards, are any of George's actions up to 1476 particularly strange, let alone indicative of mental illness or mental instability. The two major decisions he made which are often taken as such are his decision in 1470 not to side with his brother and in 1471 to change sides and go back to his brother after all. Neither of these are, however, unusual decisions for the time and they are perfectly explicable by what happened in the lead-up to 1470 and the events during the rebellion of that year. Several people did as George did, siding with the Earl of Warwick despite having originally supported Edward IV. Moreover, it is known that George's sisters and mother attempted to reconcile him with his brother, Edward. To use this as a sign of mental illness is at best cynical, at worst actively malicious, not to mention historically rather nonsensical and ignorant of the time George lived in.

George's actions of 1476 and after are, however, rather strange, and as pointed out above, even if one considers his standpoint to be correct in itself and his fears justified, they are still inexplicable. In fact, as far as can be said from a distance of over 500 years, he showed every sign that he had symptoms of paranoia,[397] a diagnosis which would make a lot of sense of his behaviour and actions, which are otherwise inexplicable, especially in the cut-throat world of fifteenth-century politics. While in that context, it would be immensely stupid to give a king suspected of trying to kill him the chance to do so legally by committing treason by accusing him of doing so, it would be a reaction that fits with the clinical pattern of paranoia. The same can be said for George's other behaviours discussed above. For any modern researcher, the evidence does suggest that George was in fact mentally ill, nor would it be surprising, given his past.

However, it is equally notable that there was no such assumption made in George's own lifetime, or even a suggestion made to that effect. While George's behaviour was considered strange, there is no suggestion it was seen as more so than that of many other traitors, such as the Earl of Warwick himself. Modern-day historians often suggest that it must have been clinical madness for George to have turned against his brother after his brother's kindness to him, but this presupposes that everything Edward said in George's attainder was indeed correct. This was definitely not the case, and contemporaries knew this. Therefore, they seemed to consider it understandable, if not very smart of George to go against him.

There is no reaction recorded to some of George's weirder and more unconventional actions, such as him openly interrupting a council meeting of Edward's to protest the execution of some of his men, which was in itself in response to George openly predicting Edward's death.[398] The existing sources portray this very calmly, almost emotionlessly.[399] While the typical somewhat outraged language usually used for treason against the king is used, it is boilerplate and there is no change made for George, neither because he was the king's brother nor because anyone seemed to consider him suffering from a mental illness. Edward, too, seemed not to consider it, as he did not spare George in any way, and did not act in any way that suggests he knew or at the very least suspected that his brother was suffering from a mental illness.

Another claim that is often made in modern history books concerned with George's behaviour and George's fate is that, apart from Edward who saw no other chance but to act as he did, his family knew that the death of George's wife had driven him over the edge. This, too, is a purely modern idea with no evidence at all to support it. The idea that his younger brother Richard, his sisters Elizabeth and Margaret and his mother Cecily Neville only protested against George's execution and pleaded for his life because they knew George could not help his behaviour is both incredibly infantilising for those suffering from mental illness and treating George as nothing more than a patient, rather than a man they loved, their brother and son. This is even notable in the language such history books have used, such as the author Matthew Lewis saying that George's brother Richard, who had protested against his execution, appeared to hold someone else responsible for his actions.[400] The implication of this is that George was only worth saving because of his mental illness, because his behaviour was supposedly influenced by that supposed mental illness, and that he would have deserved his death otherwise.

Going by the law of the fifteenth century, this is doubtlessly true. George was guilty of treason, and this meant that he had to be punished by execution. However, there were many people who were actually pardoned for treason and even for those who were not, their family often pleaded to either make his death as easy as possible, or futilely to spare them. That this would not be done for George, unless he had the excuse of suffering from mental ill-health, once more strips a person assumed to have been mentally ill of any sort of personhood beyond that. The idea that he might have been loved by his younger brother, his sisters and his mother is something that rarely seems to have been considered, something that also echoes the reporting about Henry VI in modern history books.

3.3. Modern prejudices

In Henry's case, like in George's, the idea that he might have been loved and cared for by those standing up for him and serving him, that they might have considered him not only the rightful king but one they liked, is never even brought up. In books sympathetic to him, his supporters are presented as kindly standing by him despite knowing of his unsuitability as king,[401] of not wanting to hurt a man who was not at fault for his own illness and the consequent disaster he had made of ruling the country, a man who was a kind man despite his mental illness. Books not sympathetic to him usually portray all his supporters as opportunists, those close to him as people who wanted to exploit a mentally ill man, with the idea that they might have actually liked him not even being brought up.[402] The best example for this is the shockingly hostile statement by Bertram Wolffe, who outright stated that '[i]t says much for the conservatism and restraint of the fifteenth-century English aristocracy that it took ten years from 1450 [when first Henry was called mad] before any of them ventured to propose the removal of the king himself'.[403]

A similar, if less blatant, case is George, Duke of Clarence's. Since most modern authors have decided that he was mentally unwell, he is treated to the same dismissal, if in less extreme terms. These less extreme terms are normally not because the prejudice is less than in Henry VI's case, but because his supposed mental illness is less blatant. Therefore, it cannot be treated as fact quite as much as Henry VI's illness is, and any ideas based on it are formally treated as speculation. However, it has to be pointed out that these speculations are usually rarely marked as such, the language couching them making clear that while there is no actual proof to support them, they are still correct. A classic example for this is found in John Ashdown-Hill's *The Third Plantagenet*.[404]

However, not only is there no proof for that, but there are not even any contemporary hints for it. The protestations of George's family against Edward IV's decision to have him executed are recorded. Even without looking at these records, it has to be pointed out that they had every reason to believe these protests would succeed, even without ever suspecting George was suffering from a mental illness. After all, despite there being a long and rich history of kings being betrayed by their brothers, sisters and sons, there was no precedent to them being executed, not even by kings known to have been bloodthirsty, such as Richard I of England, the so-called Lionheart. The very fact that Edward even considered it was seen as cruelty on his part, and as such the protestations of his family were only to be expected, and had nothing to do with any mental illness George may or may not have suffered from.

As it happens, there is no hint in any of the records of Cecily Neville, Dowager Duchess of York's pleas and protestations that she thought her son was in any way mentally ill. Nor is any such hint found in the pleas and protestations of George's brother Richard, Duke of Gloucester or his sisters Elizabeth, Duchess of Suffolk and Margaret, Dowager Duchess of Burgundy. Their pleas seem to have focused simply on saving George's life, imploring Edward IV to spare him because he was his brother, because they did not want him to die. Especially Richard, Duke of Gloucester is recorded to have taken his brother's death hard, and would even go on to call it 'murder by colour of law'[405] – in other words, judicial murder. Even so, however, there is no evidence that he thought George was in any way mentally unwell.

None of the language surrounding George's case gives even the slightest hint that anyone at the time thought he was mentally ill, though it did not take long for people to assume so. As early as 1550, when Raphael Holinshed wrote his *History of England*,[406] less than a century after George's death, the assumption of his suffering from a mental illness was treated as fact.

That there is little by way of evidence to judge if George actually did have a mental illness is a very interesting case for the study of how such illnesses were treated at the time, in contrast to today. In fact, in George's case it seems as if there was more tolerance for behaviour that was somewhat unusual and strange at the time than there is today, with people expressing some wonder but not actually immediately jumping to the conclusion of a mental illness.[407] George being looked at such is therefore more reflective of our society than it is of mediaeval society.

As to the question as to whether George really did suffer from clinical paranoia or some similar mental illness, or if he was mentally healthy and his behaviour simply changed after his wife's death is a question that must forever remain unanswered. Perhaps his wife was a good influence on him and ensured that he avoided such displays of temperament that he exhibited after her death, As established above, there would have been plenty of causes for George to trigger a mental illness, but the presence of such possible triggers do not prove, or even provide evidence, for an actual mental illness existing.

His behaviour could be seen to showcase symptoms of a mental illness or there might have been other reasons as to why he acted like that — a simple desire to annoy his brother, an actual grounded fear of him, a lack of proper counselling he had enjoyed until that time, and any number of other possible explanations. Which of these explanations was actually true is something that is lost to history. What if not lost is the absolutely irrevocable evidence that somewhat excessive behaviour, even somewhat inexplicable behaviour, was not immediately used as proof that someone suffered from a mental illness in the Middle Ages, and that more evidence than that was required to even make the claim. George's execution was not a popular step for Edward to take; there was a lot spoken against it[408] and according to contemporary gossip, it alienated him from his remaining family as well.[409] Had Edward seen the chance to imprison George on the grounds of insanity, to see to it he was no more danger while keeping him alive and well, it is doubtful he would not have taken that chance. Therefore, it really does seem as if this never occurred to him or any of his supporters, which once more indicates that mental illness could not be used against someone as slander, without any evidence as to the person being slandered actually suffering from some sort of mental illness. Equally, this sort of evidence had to be more than just some slightly erratic behaviour.

In fact, it is hard if not downright impossible to say just what qualified as evidence of someone suffering from a mental illness, what sort of behaviour was taken to prove it, and how it had to be qualified and quantified. We simply know that there was some sort of test in place, as this is referenced in several court cases.[410] Therefore, it is clear that such tests existed, that simply claiming it was not enough to declare someone mad and that it would be hard to use it to destroy someone's reputation.

George's death was talked about frequently in contemporary and quasi-contemporary sources, yet nobody ever suggested that he was mentally ill or even that his behaviour suggests he was mad. This was not done out of kindness towards him, his royal brother or the rest of his family because these chronicles are not overly flattering to either of them in many cases. As such, it would mean that had any of the chroniclers considered it a possibility, if not outright a fact, that George had been suffering from some sort of mental illness, they would have said so. The very fact that this was not done, that nobody said or even alluded to it, is without a doubt very telling as to what behaviour was needed to consider someone mentally ill, and that it had to be rather extreme.

In some ways, the case of George, and especially the way it was seen and treated by contemporaries, is the flipside of the same coin to the case of Juana of Castile. Whereas the latter was considered insane by all European nations upon the rumours spreading, and she was treated with hardly the barest minimum of compassion, the opposite holds true for George. His behaviour was not as extreme as Juana's was claimed to be, but nor was it normal. This did not lead to any sort of consideration of him being mad, even less to a condemnation as such, and not just in England either. Other countries reporting his execution do so while stating dry facts, and while gossip about his family's reaction and his brother Edward IV's feelings are included, no chroniclers anywhere else seemed to consider his behaviour indicative of madness or, as we would put it, mental illness, any more than George's countrymen did.

However, while this is doubtlessly interesting as it tells us what sort of behaviour was considered abnormal but by no means indicative of a mental illness, it does not allow a reverse conclusion and tell us what behaviour was, in fact, considered indicative of mental illness. What was needed to have done, or said, for how long a time period and how others had to be affected by it in order to officially class someone as mentally ill during that time is simply unknown.

Chapter 4

Religion and mental illness

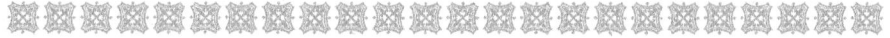

That religious aberration was punished in many ways is one of the few things almost every modern person knows, or thinks to know, about the Middle Ages. However, as will be shown in this chapter, it was not quite so easy as that, and there were many different forms of religious aberrations. Some of these were implicitly accepted by society if formally condemned,[411] such as belief in witchcraft, others were seen as heresy and punished,[412] and some of them were considered to be caused by mental illness.[413] Nor are these categories static. There are many cases in which there is an overlap, in which something that today is seen as a very clear sign of mental illness was seen either as a sign of religious enlightenment or heresy, and occasionally both.[414] On the flipside, there were cases which were seen as mental illness that would be taken as a sign of the opposite — of clear and, in fact, even bold and courageous thinking today.[415]

Cases for both have already been alluded to in the chapters above. For both of the above-mentioned theories, there are very famous examples. For the former, an example of someone who was by modern standards doubtlessly mentally ill in some way but who was seen as both a heretic and a woman chosen by God in her own lifetime is Joan of Arc. Indeed, she may be not just the most famous example in the entire Middle Ages, but quite possibly in the entirety of European history.

Joan's case has been mentioned in Chapter 2.2, but the reception to her hearing voices deserves to be looked at closely for its own sake. While due to Joan's position, it is all but impossible to see this as entirely separate from her political significance, the arguments brought when discussing her auditory hallucinations without doubt reflect the contemporary views on such phenomenon.[416] This does not mean that these arguments were not brought for political gain and with the hope of political advantages, or the fear of political disadvantages, in mind. It simply means that these arguments could not have been invented for Joan's case alone. To make such arguments work, both for and against Joan, they would have needed to have tapped into an already existing and well-established belief system.[417]

In fact, it was through this belief system that Joan first came to prominence. An old French legend told that in a time of need, a common girl, a maiden, would be chosen by God and come to save France. Obviously, with France under attack by English forces that were threatening to overrun the French, this was very definitely a time of need for France. Therefore, when Joan came to prominence, there was a readiness to believe she could be a woman who could fit the criteria and could conceivably be this woman of legend. Even so, there would need to be a sign that the woman was actually chosen by God. It could not just be any woman, but it had to be one who could in some way show evidence that she was in fact chosen by God.

By modern understanding, this is all but impossible, and the only way for it to actually work was by someone being mentally ill: either hearing voices or being otherwise so certain of her own importance and that she had been chosen by God that she could bring proof for something unprovable. For Joan, the first of these possibilities was what held true: in her own words, she heard the voices of saints telling her to save France, and she could argue her case so persuasively that she was eventually heard by the French dauphin.[418]

It has been argued that the French dauphin was so desperate he would have seized any chance to defeat the English forces and throw them out of France and given his situation this is presumably true. Even so, had he considered Joan as nothing more than mad, or even seen the chance of her actually being mad — the most natural conclusion for any modern reader when learning that someone hears voices — it is unlikely he would have given her the position he actually gave her. Such a move would have had many more dangers than they would have had merit, even allowing for the possibility that Dauphin Charles did not care that he was using a mentally ill woman for his own success.

The fact was that Joan was hardly quiet about hearing voices, and in fact used this as her justification for being in her position,[419] a position that otherwise would have been considered twice unsuited for her: because she was a woman and because she was a commoner. While commoners fought in Dauphin Charles's forces, they would not have held the position of commander, and generally, no women whatsoever were meant to fight in battle, no matter what their standing was. This flaunting of these social norms was something that would come to bite Joan later, and it would be all but impossible for Charles to go against everything that was expected of someone who was considered mentally ill. Therefore, Joan hearing voices was not actually considered a sign of madness, by him, by his men, by his troops or by his enemies.[420] Though a lot of Joan's actions were used against her once her fortunes turned, none of her enemies ever accused her of being mentally ill and her hearing voices were never used against her as such. Her claims seemed to be totally accepted, it was only the meaning behind these voices that was questioned and with mental illness not being considered even a possibility due to the rather strict belief set of the Middle Ages, which actually encompassed hearing voices as a sign of either God or the devil. Even in the centuries after her death, this was never used against Joan. Not even William Shakespeare, in his questionably at times historic plays, stated she was 'mad', though madness was something the playwright used often and famously. Instead, he stated she was a witch and in league with the devil, something that her enemies also used against her contemporarily.[421]

The fact that she heard voices therefore singled her out somewhat, but saw her neither ostracised nor elevated above others. It was only when she could prove that these voices said something that not only Dauphin Charles but a whole panel of clergymen considered to be religiously sound that she was considered to possibly be the woman legend spoke of. Even that was not enough; poor Joan also had to endure an embarrassing procedure by which it was checked if she was actually a virgin, as the woman of legend who was to save France in its time of need was said to be. Only once it was clear she fulfilled all these criteria was she taken seriously as the maiden of legend.

What would have happened had she not managed to fulfil all criteria is unknown and guesswork, but the presence of churchmen to check her answers suggests that if not, she would have landed in trouble with the

Church. Obviously, the idea of her being a fraud floated, as did the idea of her being led astray by the devil, but the idea of the voices she heard being but a figment of her imagination, a hallucination brought on by some sort of mental illness, was not.[422]

The English against whom she fought had a very similar take on Joan and the voices she heard as did the French, only diametrically opposed, as of course their aims were diametrically opposed. Joan hearing voices that helped the French defeat the English forces were thought to be inspired by God himself;[423] to actually be the saints that Joan said were speaking to her. For the English, it was equally obviously inspired by the devil; demons giving Joan advice to accomplish something God himself would never want.

What seems to have been a theory that was addressed by the men who tried Joan once she was captured by the English and had to stand trial, was that she was in fact only pretending to hear voices,[424] that she used the idea of saints speaking to her as a way to sneak herself into a position not rightfully hers, a position God had not intended for her. Again, this shows a set of religious beliefs that stand in stark contrast to medical knowledge of the twentieth and twenty-first centuries. Nowadays, claiming to hear voices would only convince everyone that someone was suffering from a mental illness, while in the fifteenth century, religion dictated that it was a sign from either God or the devil, and that claiming to hear saints could actually lead to a prestigious position.[425]

Pretending to hear voices, however, was often considered blasphemy, and was, as such, all but unheard of.[426] There are several typical cases, which will be discussed below. So an initial suspicion that Joan may have been pretending she could hear voices was not unusual and hardly far-fetched. Upon Joan not falling for any trick questions, however, and thus there being no proof that she was actually pretending, or even that she received voices from the devil, a rather mean trick had to be used to see to it Joan could be executed for heresy after all.

Just what voices Joan actually heard, how this manifested, if she did indeed pretend and if not, what it was she suffered from, are questions that can no longer be answered. Even so, it is obvious that it was religion, rather than medicine, which was thought to answer the question as to why she could hear voices nobody else could hear. One of the most blatant symptoms of mental illness for modern-day people was not even connected with mental health, and lack thereof, at the time. If Joan actually heard voices, then she must have suffered from some sort of mental illness, but what it was and how it manifested there is no way of saying. It is only clear that it was considered to be a religious matter, nothing else, and it depended on what these voices said as to whether someone was seen as religiously enlightened, chosen by God Himself, or led astray by the devil. The cures for these also depended on what version was considered more likely in every individual case.

In the case of someone being believed, and themselves convinced, to be hearing voices from God, there was usually no treatment of any sort offered. In these cases it was seen as something good, and actually would be considered a punishment if the voices went away, rather than the other way around. Though it could sometimes turn into outright delusions, which caused those suffering from them to perform actions that could be harmful to them, as long as they were considered to be coming from God or the saints, these actions were not considered a sign of madness.[427] On the contrary, there are several cases recorded in which such actions were actually seen as a sign of a particular piety and praised as such; seen as a reason as to why the person was hearing the voices in the first place. Since this often included extreme self-harm, with the wearing of hairshirts perhaps as one of the least harmless examples, this usually caused extreme physical discomfort, something which is known to strengthen the symptoms of mental illness. These special cases, therefore, would have only gone towards making auditory hallucinations worse. In short, it would have been a vicious circle, with religion standing actively in the way of recovery, or even recognition of the problem. Presenting it as desirable could, and in some cases, did, in fact, lead to death by encouraging those suffering from mental illness to listen to the voices in their head and causing them to believe that this was actually good for them, if not physically then for the good of their soul.[428]

If the voices were, however, considered to be the work of the devil, everything was different and getting rid of them was a priority. In itself, that would be a good thing. Even if these symptoms were not treated as part of a mental illness but instead as a sort of religious sickness, this would doubtlessly have helped in some way. However, both the stigma attached to it and the cures used against it would definitely not have helped.

There was a lot more stigma attached to hearing voices that were considered religiously impure (to be actively influenced by the devil or demons) than there was to being simply mentally ill, such as Henry VI and Charles VI were. While, as has been discussed above, mental illnesses were often not treated much differently than physical illnesses were, and there was often not much more stigma attached,[429] this was different when it was believed that the devil was at work. If someone suffered from a mental illness that was not actually recognised as such and it was seen as a sign of, at best, the devil's perfidy, at worst as a sign of the extreme sinfulness of the sufferer, it was often considered to have been started by some religious misbehaviour. Conversely, sometimes the symptoms were recognised as being part of a mental illness, but it was considered to have been brought on by religious misbehaviour.

In the case of the former, of someone hearing voices that were considered to have been either caused by the devil or to be demons or the devil, there was not only the stigma attached and the social ramifications to be considered, but it would also lead to self-loathing. The treatments for this were pretty gruesome as well. Naturally, a lot of ideas, of treatments and cures, even for the most harmless physical sickness, sound gruesome to modern ears while they were considered perfectly normal at the time and were not thought to be in any way terrible or even a punishment. However, the treatment for hearing voices caused by the devil were not only considered terrible at the time, but they were actually deliberately painful.[430] These treatments included physical torture, punishments that were otherwise used on criminals and even then, were looked at with disgust by most people. Other treatments were actually designed to make the person sick, to thus drive the devil, demons, or whatever other malignant spirits were thought to inhabit the stricken person, out. The theory was that the devil and his demons preferred to attack healthy people, so as to be able to cause more mischief.[431] Therefore, to weaken the person thus suffering was often meant to be an exercise in driving any bad influences away. At the same time, it was meant to strengthen the spirit of the person so afflicted, to give them more mental power of resistance. By this logic, the physical mistreatment that constituted treatment for the voices was a treatment for the mind, so to speak, that was meant to stabilise the mind until the devil, demons or other malignant spirits had no more point of attack.[432]

These treatments often included being made to vomit; in fact purging in general, to get the devil to be expelled in this way. Though it was not an actual exorcism as the word and practice is understood today, it worked very similarly. In fact, it sometimes killed people, which was seen as a sad conclusion, but one that was considered better than continuing to be used by the devil.[433]

The consequence was that mentally ill people were targeted specifically, and specifically due to their symptoms, to endure cruel punishments that could even result in death. This was done to 'cure' them of symptoms often thought, or at least implicitly assumed, to have been their fault.[434] Though the opposite did happen and in some cases mentally ill people were considered to be particularly pious, it does seem that for this to be considered, there needed to be a certain proof that the voices being heard were those of saints, which was hard. Though in the case of it being considered the opposite, it was understood that a cure was necessary, but it was not a cure designed to stop mental illnesses, but something else entirely, a demonic possession which was seen as a separate issue from actual mental illnesses.

In fact, it might come from these stories, stressed during the Renaissance, that our modern-day image of how mentally ill people were treated during the Middle Ages comes from. Many of the myths passed down the centuries have a smidgeon of truth that explicitly come from the treatment of people who had one of the most classic symptoms of mental illness: those who heard voices that could not be heard by anyone else.

In some ways, everything these prejudices say about mediaeval 'mental health care', such as it was, is exactly what can be seen in how these people were treated. Sometimes even subjected to torture, their death was considered collateral damage to save their souls,[435] and especially that it was the Church behind all this. The one theory that can be debunked, even so, is the idea of this treatment being deliberate, designed only to hurt people for being mentally ill. As can be seen in Joan of Arc's case, at the time, hearing voices in itself was not considered a sign of mental illness.[436] It was considered a religious sign and certainly an all-powerful Church who wanted to punish mentally ill people for their condition would not seize only on this one symptom and declare it to be a religious sign, while leaving all the other signs of mental illness (which, as discussed above, were well-known and treated with at least a modicum of compassion) out of the equation.[437]

Instead, it is simply that due to lack of understanding of this issue, clergymen, as much as anyone one else, actually believed that it was a religious sign and also considered that the best way to treat this was by applying the horrifying cures discussed in Chapter 2. Though it is perfectly possible that there were those who enjoyed administering such pain, and who did not believe that this helped but still did it, the evidence for that is scant. What evidence there is suggests that this was actually what was believed by everyone involved, clergymen, priests and others associated with the Church as much as those afflicted with hearing voices and their relatives, and that the treatment given to them was considered nasty but necessary. The very fact that even clergymen so stricken also were subjected to such treatments, with no difference between them and patients who were laymen,[438] also does not suggest that there was some far-reaching scheme to be evil and target mentally ill people for the fun of it by the mediaeval Church, to terrorise everyone into submission.

Even so, the fact that they really believed it must have been poor comfort for those stricken with a mental illness that made them hear voices, and the terrible treatment meted out to some patients cannot be denied. An even darker subject is a mental illness associated with religious doubts. For this, the best example is Juana of Castile, whose case is mentioned above.

Juana had the bad luck of being born to famously religious-intolerant parents, who actively persecuted everyone of a different religion than their own very strict and unforgiving Catholicism. It is, in fact, one of the things Isabella of Castille and Ferdinand of Aragon are most famous for, that earned them the nickname 'the Catholic Monarchs'[439] and in this case, the public association is not mistaken. Most famously, perhaps, they ordered all Jewish citizens to either convert or leave their lands and demanded from their son-in-law he do the same. Though this was not unheard of — Edward I had done the same in England some centuries earlier[440] — it was rather uncommon at the time, with most monarchs stressing their own Catholicism but being much less extreme and tolerating Jewish and Muslim citizens.

In some ways, of course, actions such as those undertaken by Isabella and Ferdinand were populist, but in their case, we know it went way beyond that. Their extreme piety and belief in every word the Catholic Church uttered by their bishops and the Pope started one of the darkest and most brutal chapters in Church history: the Spanish Inquisition.

Whole books have been written about this and the history of it. The Catholic Monarchs' contribution to, or even their very idea of, its founding and the details of it have been discussed elsewhere. It is not the intention of this book to go over this familiar territory again but to show what the sort of culture and family, especially, that Juana of Castile was born into was like.

There was absolutely no tolerance of any even slightly different belief in Spain at that time,[441] which was unfortunate for poor Juana, who was not only critical of her parents' beliefs and ideas, but seems to have been at least somewhat doubtful of the Church's dogma in general.[442]

It is actually debated if Juana's recorded mental illness was brought on by how her parents and, under their instruction, the Church reacted to her doubts,[443] if her doubts were in fact seen as evidence of her suffering from a mental illness in itself,[444] or if the way she made these doubts known was somewhat erratic or unusual.[445] However, it seems that her parents at the very least thought that her refusal to believe all they believed, and her refusal to give into it no matter how they tried to 'treat' this, was evidence of mental illness.

Shockingly, it seems that the concept of a 'cure' for what Isabella and Ferdinand believed, or at the very least pretended to believe, was a mental illness seemed to be to torture their daughter into submission, until her will broke.[446] The suggestion is that they did not care for her physical wellbeing, or even for her mental wellbeing, as long as she was religiously in tune with them.[447] Though some of what was done to Juana can only be guessed at, there are stories of her being hanged by her wrists by chains from the ceiling,[448] one of the torture methods later used by the Spanish Inquisition, and one that often in fact led to death.[449] The only concern of Juana's mother, Isabella, upon this being done to her daughter, however, was that she did not recant her beliefs and thus did not give up what Isabella considered her 'madness'.[450] This is perhaps the best indicator that Juana's mental illness was in fact at first nothing but having an open and doubting mind towards religion and not falling in line with her parents' extremist views.[451] Later, as has been discussed above, she had stronger symptoms, symptoms that even today can be seen as being indicative of mental illness, but this does not have to mean that Juana's parents were right from the beginning in considering her to be 'mad'. Her mental illness could very well have been caused by the childhood trauma of being tortured by her parents and the Church she was supposed to believe in, for not agreeing with them.

There is nothing that can be said in defence of this. It has been pointed out that it is possible that Isabella and Ferdinand quite legitimately believed that their daughter's refusal to believe what they so strongly believed in was a mental illness, but even so, this was not the typical behaviour towards those who were mentally ill.[452] Isabella and Ferdinand were ruthless; they would have known exactly what harm, physically and mentally, torture methods such as were used on Juana could have on someone. They still not only agreed to have it done to their daughter but actively encouraged it.[453] It can be seen as an attempt to break her will, an attempt, in short, to bring on a legitimate mental illness to see to it their daughter stopped believing something they did not approve of.

Especially during the time of the Spanish Inquisition, Juana's case was hardly the only one, though hers is the most famous one. In the history of the Spanish Inquisition, there are many similar cases, of people who were considered mentally ill for not believing in the very strict belief system of the mediaeval Spanish Church,[454] a belief system that, in fact, was much worse than in the centuries before and also much stricter, at least for the time being, than it was in other countries around Spain.[455] Much of the torture was explicitly because of this, to make those who did not share the same belief system submit. This has caused the idea that, in fact, mental illnesses were hated so much that torture was not only accepted but encouraged, and that all those who were mentally ill were in fact tortured, ostracised and punished throughout the Middle Ages. This is presumably also why there is a belief that this was the same for any and all mental illness they suffered from. In fact, what seems to have happened was that mental illness was used as an excuse; it was not that those who were mentally ill were immediately tortured, harmed and in many cases killed to be cured, but that those who did not believe in the strict belief system set by the Church were declared mentally ill, the very lack of belief considered its own mental illness, and the torture considered its treatment, which was naturally only a way to get those who were a danger to those ideas to submit.[456] That this ended in actual mental illness and death was then considered a cure of sorts, or at the very least, a kind of collateral damage.

It is hard, if not downright impossible, to say whether those who used these arguments actually believed in them, or used them as an excuse to mistreat others, as it is always hard, if not impossible, to say that those following a system that ostracises those who believe differently actually believe such arguments or instead use them as an excuse.

This would seem to indicate that in this case, all the stereotypes, the myths and the prejudices against mediaeval people and the way they treated mental illnesses were justified. This is both true and not true. It is true in the way that there had to be an excuse found to torture those who did not agree to submit. The Spanish Inquisition, a system that was meant to harm and suppress all those who did not believe the same, had absolutely no problem with harming, hurting and killing Jewish people, Muslim people and generally everyone who was not Christian, simply for not being Christian, and this was the only explanation that was needed. However, this could not be used for Christians who were more tolerant, who technically believed in all the Church said, but in a less fundamentalist, extremist way.[457] Since all such systems need the support of people to be able to work and as such, could not simply imprison Christians who were not dehumanised the way everyone non-Christian was, there needed to be an excuse. Mental illness was the excuse used, though it is very obvious that none of the people responsible for it considered it a legitimate mental illness. Perhaps, like Ferdinand and Isabella, they believed that disagreement actually was a mental illness, and that it was dangerous for body and soul. Even so, there can be no doubt that there would have been an awareness of the consequences of the treatment meted out to them. As a matter of fact, in some ways, this makes the whole concept of how these people were 'treated' even more horrifying. If someone actually believed a person was mentally ill for disagreeing, and their solution was to subject them to treatment that could and frequently did see people killed, this shows a callousness that is hard to put into words.

Curiously, it also goes against other evidence we have of how mental illnesses were regarded and how they were treated, in other places, which is what makes this case relevant for this study. In late mediaeval England, it was widely known that mental illness could and did make the sufferers unable to think straight and therefore often say things that were considered dangerous, even blasphemous under different circumstances.[458] Such statements did not usually go unpunished, and in fact, punishments were often quite embarrassing.[459] However, if it could be proved that the person having said it was mentally ill, there was no such punishment.[460] Usually, it ended in them being treated for the mental illness, in ways that were not exactly pleasant but that were not designed to be hurtful and the end result of which was meant to be a cure, not a broken will and mindless submission. In many ways, treatment of the mentally ill was therefore the very opposite of that which was meted out by the Spanish Inquisition, and, as such, was horrifying even to many contemporaries. Even if the Inquisitors did believe they were actually treating truly mentally ill people, that religious lack of compliance could not be explained in any other way, their behaviour can be neither explained nor excused. It is simply inexcusable.

This, of course, once more suggests that mental illness, or at least some sort of mental illness, were stigmatised to the point of there being no protests if those said to be suffering from it were tortured, sometimes even to death. Whether this is actually true is hard to find out, but definitely, the suggestion is underlying. There are, though, four facts that have to be taken into account when judging this, while keeping the utter inhumanity of the proceedings in mind.

The first of these facts is that the Spanish Inquisition and those following its lead worked with terror. This means that while there was supposed to be a sort of support from the general population at some point, it was achieved by fear and terror, by scaring many into submission and hurting those who did not. Just how much this was a part of the acceptance of what was done to Christians, to the people singled out as mentally ill, is hard to say. It may have been a significant part, or it may not. It is quite as possible that similar to the Jewish population and the Muslim population, those who were singled out as mentally ill were simply otherised to the point that there was an 'us versus them' mentality, and that this contributed largely to the widespread acceptance, or at least, the widespread ignorance of what was happening.

The second important fact is that the mental illness that the Spanish Inquisition targeted was in fact mostly invented. Perfectly healthy people who simply did not agree with their beliefs were declared mentally ill explicitly because of that, and then subjected to horrifying treatments. Other mental illnesses were not.[461] There is no evidence that illnesses such as paranoia or depression were particularly targeted or cruelly treated, though undoubtedly there was more fear of any of these illnesses slipping into something that could be taken as religious disagreement and as such, would once more putting the sufferers in danger of falling foul of the religious instances of the radicalised Church.[462] In itself, however, there was no danger inherent in these mental illnesses, and they were not stigmatised any more than at any other time, and any other illness.

Another important fact is that some physical illnesses were also stigmatised and in fact seen as evidence of God's wrath and thus punished.[463] Not all of them were, and many physical illnesses, like mental ones, were mainly ignored, with no outside threats of danger. Others were treated as a sign of someone's sinfulness. Therefore, there was obviously a danger in not being healthy in general, which is horrible but somehow takes the immediate stress away from mentally ill people as a primary target as this was simply not true.

The last fact, though, illuminates the flipside and suggests that otherising people suffering from anything than less than perfect health was part of how the Inquisition managed to act as they did, and that they did it with the complete support of Isabella and Ferdinand, their support even extending to the mistreatment of their own daughter. That, however, an organisation so famously intolerant, so keen on catching anyone who might have even mildly differing religious opinions, had to resort to calling some of those they wanted to force into submission mentally ill is a rather terrible reflection not only on them but on late mediaeval Spanish society as a whole. The Spanish Inquisition was not usually known for mincing words or considering the feelings of anyone, but there must have been a fear that it would not be acceptable to hurt people like Juana simply for having mildly differing opinions. It has been suggested that Juana was the only such case, that all others sharing her opinions were simply arrested and tortured for blasphemy or disagreement, but this is not the case. Certainly, it would have been hard under any circumstances to torture Juana, except in the one the poor girl found herself in, with her parents enthusiastically supporting it. Under these circumstances, there would have been no need to invent a reason for her treatment, but simply being a blasphemer would have done well. She found herself in the same circumstances as those of lower birth who found themselves on the wrong side of the Inquisition.

In other words, there was a fear, and quite possibly, given what we actually do know, a grounded fear that arresting devout Christians for blasphemy was not something that would have been accepted, or at least something that would have caused an uproar. Doing the same to mentally ill people was not feared to cause any trouble, and in the event, it didn't.

There is no beating around the bush in this instance: mentally ill people were not considered as important as those who were healthy, and this very lethargy towards them was used to target and victimise people. In short, though many of those so arrested were not actually mentally ill, it was only made possible, or only made possible in the form it was, because of the way mentally unhealthy people were ostracised.[464]

This seems to indicate that the attitude towards mental health and mental illnesses was rather different in southern Europe than in England, France and, at least at the time, the Holy Roman Empire. This, too, is suggested by evidence, so that it makes a very coherent if utterly gruesome picture.

In conclusion, the evidence in this case suggests that mental illness was indeed hugely stigmatised and that this very stigma was used to justify maltreatment not only of those who were actually mentally ill, but it enabled maltreatment of political and religious enemies on the charge of them being mentally ill. This, even more than the horrifying treatments of those who heard voices and could not prove that these voices were of saints or God, is presumably also where most of the ideas about mental illness in mediaeval times comes from: the stigma, the otherisation, the dehumanisation, the terrible treatment, the callousness with which side effects from maltreatment, up to and including death, were regarded. All of this is found in the time of the Spanish Inquisition in southern Europe, and therefore is legitimately part of the treatment of mentally ill people during the time of the Middle Ages. It is, however, hardly the only part. Other aspects, and far better treatment, far kinder assumptions about mentally ill people, have been discussed above. For this chapter, it is interesting that nor is it the only aspect of religion and mental illness, or even, for most of the Middle Ages and most of Europe, the most common treatment.

This is quite understandable of course. The Middle Ages cover a long period of time and Europe consisted of several very different nations with very different cultures. That things changed through the years and across the regions is only logical. However the assumption that the treatment meted out by the Church to mentally ill people during the time of the Spanish Inquisition (and the disregard with which mentally ill people were in fact treated by them by using mental illness as an excuse) often leads people to reach the conclusion that there was constant mistreatment of mentally ill people by the Church.

But this is not the case, and there is also lot of evidence to suggest differing treatments of those suffering from mental illness by clergymen. We can therefore form a much more varied picture of the Church's attitude towards mental illness, one that differs across the regions during the Middle Ages, and across cultures during several different centuries.

During the Spanish Inquisition, the worst of humanity was showcased by those religiously Christian, not only towards those suffering from a mental illness of course, but also, more famously, towards anyone who did not share their very strict, dogmatic beliefs. Opposed to that, in some ways, there were also churchmen who showed the very best of humanity in their treatment of those sick, including those who were mentally ill, during the Middle Ages.

Perhaps most famously, and the most widely known instance of this is the fact that monasteries and convents were not just a place of learning, nor simply a place of debauchery as they are so often portrayed today, and as they have been portrayed since the Renaissance. Very significantly, they were also hospitals; hospitals that did not charge like Bedlam Hospital did but which accepted everyone, free of charge, and took care of them.[465] Most usually, if this is at all alluded to in works about mediaeval medicine, these hospitals are presented as being for physical illnesses, the way modern hospitals are, with mentally ill patients being ignored.[466] This was not, however, the reality of monasteries and convents throughout the Middle Ages, in England as well as the Holy Roman Empire, Scotland, France and what is today Italy. Monasteries and convents being a place for people to be taken care of and cured, who had no other place to go, were a very widespread idea, and in fact, one of the tenets of Christianity, and therefore also of the Church itself. Though this was only a theory and not always, or even very often, practised, it is still notable that it was one of the core ideas of Christianity and, as such, often also preached.

There is sadly not much by way of evidence as to how these hospitals were run by nuns and monks, but there is much commentary on them,[467] observations that are directly opposed to most people's ideas of the Middle Ages and the supposedly dehumanising treatment given to everyone but the most healthy of people at the time.

Most of the comments made about these hospitals refer to physical health, but there is evidence that these hospitals were just as open for mentally ill patients. Some evidence for this is the language in general used about such hospitals, which wildly veered between admiration and disgust, with both being a reflection on whatever the person in question thought about illness (physical and mental) and how they wished to see them treated. In general, it seems that there was a lot of gratitude for these free hospitals and that they were accessible to anyone.[468] Naturally, there would be a religious factor involved, but it is not true, as is often assumed, that the belief system of the time was that illness was God-given and that treatment was therefore not allowed because it interfered with God's plans. This is an idea for which there is little evidence at any time during the Middle Ages, for any place in Europe. While illness, like most other events, was considered either as God-given or caused by the devil, there is no contemporary source that states that those stricken, with any physical or mental illness, should not be treated or that God Himself would object to that. For mental illnesses this argument is made particularly often, but it is not any truer than it is for physical illnesses. There was only one area for which this counted, and that was when someone was born mentally ill in some way or had some illness that made them unable to function like most of society. In this case, though, it was not considered to be a punishment, a test if those so stricken could stand this test given to them by God, but instead their illnesses were simply seen as a fact of life. The fact of it being God-given was more that such people should not be a victim of prejudice, as sadly they tended to be even more often than today, but that they should be seen as children of God just as much as anyone else. God had chosen to make them different, but it was not a flaw, not something wrong, simply another divine choice that humans had to accept.

In some ways, such ideas show the exact opposite of the attitude exhibited during the Spanish Inquisition. Whereas during that time, prejudice against mentally ill people was stoked and could then be used against anyone so afflicted, with the accusation of mental illness used as explanation as to why people had to be tortured, this attitude not only showed a far softer attitude but actually outright demanded the opposite — declaring prejudice against those suffering from mental illness or any other illness, to be directly against God's wishes. Rather than seeing those afflicted as having to be violently suppressed and 'cured' if someone was a bit unusual, if someone suffered from a mental illness, it was considered to be God's wish for those people to be different, to not fit exactly into society, and for their minds to work differently than those of most people.[469]

These were not just empty words. Especially in villages where everyone tended to know everyone else, clergymen actually went out of their way to make life as easy as possible for people stricken with a mental illness, for people whose mental state did not make it easy for them to fit into society, and to smooth their path in life. Often, such men and women were employed by the Church,[470] to be a useful part of society as best as they could, while not demanding of them to conform to expectations they could not have fulfilled. That this was helpful is not only common sense, but actually confirmed. Studies over the past decades have showed that ever since authority figures such as priests and clergymen have stopped holding an elevated position, and begun to help members of society who might be suffering from a mental illness by using their authority to protect them from prejudices, life was, or could be, more difficult for those who were not under such protection.

Naturally, the fact that priests had such power, power that especially in small villages often ran unchecked, could cause immense problems. and there was a lot of abuse of this power. There is, however, no evidence that throughout the Middle Ages, there was more abuse of priestly power than any other power, and there is evidence that in some ways, the Church was a force for good, especially for those suffering from mental illness.

It was not just that the Church offered hospitals in which those suffering from mental illness could be treated, and that many of those in power actively helped men and women suffering from mental illnesses. The monasteries and convents did not just have hospitals to help those suffering from an illness, they were in fact a sanctuary for all who needed it. For example, it is often assumed nowadays that the Church only wanted 'perfect' humans to show they were made in the image of God, and therefore anyone else was rejected.[471] This is said, for example, in many leaflets from the Enlightenment.[472] The opposite is the case; monasteries and convents were, in the words of several popes,[473] often the places where the outcasts of society, the unwanted, the uncared for, found their home along with compassion and affection. Though, as has been established above, it would be wrong to see mentally ill people as outcasts of society even then, in many cases, they were still considered to be an embarrassment for the family, particularly if the person stricken with illness was an heir, someone who was meant to, but was unable to inherit possessions.

That these men, and, more rarely, women, went to monasteries and convents does not only have an explanation of piety and religious compassion, but had a more practical reason: this was the only way that a younger brother, or even a younger sister (through her husband) could inherit what was originally meant to go to their elder sibling.[474] Since religious vocation was an accepted reason for not fulfilling the expected duties of an heir, and moreover eased the way for a younger sibling to step into their shoes, there was often little choice but to have a mentally ill son or brother become a monk. In such cases, the acceptance of monasteries, and more rarely convents, of such mentally ill men or women was rarely caused simply by compassion. Often, rich and noble parents would give the monastery or convent a sizeable amount of money or a part of their lands to have their sons or daughters become a monk or nun. However, there is no evidence that there was more money involved if a mentally unwell person entered such an institution.

In other cases, when an inheritance wasn't involved, it was still an act of compassion for monks and nuns to accept someone into their midst who was unable to take care of him- or herself and who was mentally ill. Often, this was done with the intention of giving these outcast men or women the best home as well as the best care that was possible, and as such, it was a very good option for many.

There is, of course, always the underlying assumption that the people who took this option did so because of a lack of other options; because of the difficulties of living in the world their families inhabited, a world that was not made for people who had mental illnesses and could often be actively hostile to them. That this is not entirely correct, at least for most of the Middle Ages and most of the places in Europe, has amply been proven in Chapters 1 and 3. It was not only possible but not even uncommon for those said to suffer from mental illnesses to still be able to function in society. For logical reasons, we only have explicit examples from the nobility, such as George Latimer's case. Despite having been declared to suffer from 'idiocy', there was nothing that was stopping him from participating in society, and though his brother took over the management of his lands, this did not mean that George had nothing left to do. On the contrary, it was probably meant to make life easier for him and as such, enable him to live the best life he could, despite his 'idiocy'. That this was not just possible on paper is shown by what happened to William Beaumont, who could and did continue living in the society that is so freely claimed to have ostracised people like him simply for suffering from a mental illness. Despite not managing his own lands, he was able to do as he pleased, with little or no control, otherwise there would have been no reason for him to eventually be stripped of this as well, to be declared to be unable to do so. Obviously, if he had already been controlled tightly, there would have been no reason for him to behave in a way that could in some way reflect badly on the king, whatever this means in detail.

It could be argued that the cases of Lord Latimer and Viscount Beaumont are not representative of society as a whole since they were wealthy and influential nobles. This is doubtlessly possible, but there is no evidence to contradict the notion of it being any different in the lower echelons of society. Therefore, all we do have suggests that society as a whole was much more accepting of mentally ill people and could accommodate them perfectly well, with no explicit evidence to the contrary. While it can therefore be argued that it must have been different, it is nothing but speculation, contradicting the evidence we have.

Therefore, joining a monastery or convent may not have been simply the only option even for poor people when suffering from a mental illness. It does seem to have been the best option, however, for a variety of reasons. First, in many cases, the people who made this decision had lost their family; a sad fate that was in fact not just restricted to mentally ill people who joined a monastery or convent. Many poor people did make the decision exactly for those reasons and it was especially widespread for those who suffered from an illness, physical or mental. In fact, this was so common that it was remarked upon contemporarily all through the Middle Ages.

There is no suggestion that anyone considering such a decision felt they had no other options; many, in fact, considered it to be a very good option. Religious communities were known to have been inclusive and while that doesn't in itself mean that outside society was exclusive (which has been analysed in depth in Chapters 1 and 3) there were necessities of life which stopped society as a whole from being as inclusive as such small communities in monasteries and convents were.

This had nothing to do with discrimination towards those suffering from mental illness. Discrimination did exist, as has been shown above, but the unsuitability of society for many of those suffering from both physical and mental illness was not deliberate. And it is here that we see the real difference between nobles and commoners. The necessities of life meant that for commoners, it was much harder to exist in society with some form of mental illness. Unlike nobles, who were very wealthy and whose work mostly comprised managing their lands with more or less involvement, most commoners had to work to survive. There were systems in place, systems of neighbourly help if someone was injured and could not work for a while, ways of taking care of those who could not take care of themselves, but even so, it could become rather difficult for someone who would not be able, due to physical or mental illness, to ever take care of themselves or their own family.[475] Especially if they had lost their own family, it was simply easier for many to become a monk or nun than try and earn money in a world that was not suited for those who had a more severe form of mental illness to work.[476]

By becoming a monk or nun, not only were there no more worries about having enough money for their upkeep, enough money not to starve, there was also another perk, something that even modern-day psychologists know is of much help for many forms of mental illness: a steady routine.[477] This is something convents and monasteries are well known for even today, and it is the one idea about mediaeval religious institutions which is entirely correct: they were very organised and every day was well structured.

This, explicitly, is known to have helped many of those who entered a monastery. But there was one special subgroup of mentally ill people, especially, who found comfort in these daily routines: those who were, in modern terms, shell-shocked by experiences in battles and wars, or traumatised by such experiences.

As has been alluded to above, it is often claimed today that shell-shock is a mental health issue that has only been discovered after the First World War, and then only because so very many men, from all corners of society, were affected. This is not entirely untrue; certainly, that was when most people became aware of it, when it became a widespread subject and awareness soared. The very name used for this phenomenon, 'shell-shock', alludes to when it was first examined and taken very seriously.[478]

However, while it was only then that this sort of trauma received a closer look by doctors at large, and was examined and named, the ailment itself has been around for a long time. In the Middle Ages, it seems as if it was simply seen as one form of trauma. Trauma itself was already widely known at the time and taken quite seriously. It was well understood by priests accompanying soldiers, for example, and there are records of men being stricken with it, of being unable to fight due to it, as well as of women losing their children and showing signs of what we today would call trauma.[479]

As has been discussed above, there was even knowledge that events that were common and that most people could and did survive without any difficulties could cause mental illnesses in others, and that this was treated with compassion, with the understanding that the person so stricken was simply not made for life in the ways others were. In such cases, it was often the people so affected themselves who made the decision to enter a monastery or convent, and the regularity of the days and the structure of monastery life really appealed to traumatised people.[480]

Today we would not classify trauma as a mental illness. However, we do know it can lead to mental illnesses on occasion, and we also know that during the Middle Ages, it was considered a form of mental illness. It was also understood, though, that the structure and the simplicity of life in a convent or monastery helped.

Once more, to understand this, we have to dismiss our modern notions of life in a convent or monastery, notions that are badly coloured by Renaissance and Reformation ideas, explicitly created to defame both the Middle Ages and such Church institutions. Due to these perceptions, and also due to a lot of our own modern structures, it is easy to believe that monasteries and convents were not only massively rich organisations, but that they were full of monks and nuns gorging themselves, keeping to no rule at all, having orgies and committing other sins that they openly preached against. We may even have been led to believe that they took extra joy in doing not only what they forbade but what they actively punished others for doing.[481]

Much of this depiction is political propaganda and, sadly, it is still repeated as fact by many, even in books that proclaim to be non-fiction.[482]

As with everything, this is not to say that this was always untrue. There were monasteries and convents that were less than devout, and even ones that at the same time preached against sins with particular vigour. These examples should, however, not be taken as the norm. As ever, since these monasteries and convents were run by humans, there were human flaws. Depending on who was in charge, they may have been more or less equipped for dealing with the behaviour of their monks and nuns or taken more or less interest in the problems of society. If the person who was in charge did not have any especial interest in being too pious, then rules and structures would not be followed, and perhaps sins the Church usually preached against, such as fornication and gluttony, were encouraged and the problems of the society around them ignored.[483] It differed from case to case, but what evidence there is suggests that most of these institutions were as pious and as caring as they were meant to be.

Many such institutions therefore took in the outcasts of society, the members of society who, through no fault of their own had difficulties fitting into mediaeval society. Those suffering from mental illness were a perfect example for that. Even the sort of mental illness that could be ostracised in society, such as hearing voices thought to have been caused by the devil, was, if not accepted, certainly not judged as badly inside convents and monasteries as it was elsewhere. This is quite possibly because it was considered that giving your life to God and attempting to serve him in all you did was the best way to get rid of any demonic influences. The treatments given for this were also much less harsh in convents and monasteries than they were elsewhere, with the main treatment appearing to be silence and prayer.[484]

This may not have helped as much as many modern pharmaceutical solutions can, but given the treatments available at the time for the mentally ill, prayers and silence may have been the best option; the best hope for betterment of the condition there was. It would certainly have been better than many of the gruesome suggestions given by priests to laypersons, who were still meant to deal with the world. These treatments, discussed above, would in most cases have exacerbated the condition rather than cure it or at least lessen the symptoms. This could not be said for prayers and silence. Even if it did not help, it would not actively make a condition worse.

Perhaps most importantly of all, though, was that unless someone was so mentally ill that they were unaware of their surroundings and unable to participate in daily life, that everyone in a convent and monastery was made to feel like a valuable member of society by the monks and nuns.[485] In most cases, the monasteries and nunneries were genuinely devoted to bettering those that were part of its community as well as society at large. This meant that unlike in secular society, where even if the best efforts were taken, someone who, due to a mental illness, could not do the same work as others, could not contribute the way others did and might therefore feel rather left out, could feel just as valuable a part of the community as everyone else.

We have a particularly valuable primary source to illustrate this, from the twelfth-century nun, Hildegard von Bingen. Very famous for having written down several helpful recipes (even by modern standards) for medicine against an array of ailments,[486] she herself suffered from what we today know must have been a mental illness: she too heard voices.[487] These voices were, particularly after her death, considered to have come from saints and were therefore not stigmatised or even considered to be a mental illness, but it is known that she herself struggled with it, and that not everyone, not even everyone in her community, accepted her.[488] Some arguments held with her escalated, to the point where one particular case was taken to the Pope.[489] The point being made, apparently, was that Hildegard was not suited to be an abbess; not that she should be ostracised completely but just not be part of the community as a whole.[490]

Perhaps most tellingly, the Pope, and most of Hildegard's fellow nuns, did not agree.[491] The case against her failed, meaning that someone suffering from a mental illness, and actually struggling with it in her lifetime, could not only become a valuable member of society in a convent, but also hold some power there. Not only that, but it was supported and actively encouraged by the Pope that Hildegard, a woman suffering from a mental illness, should be allowed that sort of power.

Hildegard being an abbess also gives us a very good idea of what sorts of powers were given to her, and thereby what sort of powers could be given to someone who was mentally ill. Some, if not all of her symptoms were considered alarming by her peers but trust was placed in her by most of her community despite this.[492] The fact was that bringing up those symptoms with the Pope was seen as slander and that it was not, by many people, considered a sensible reason to exclude her from the position of abbess or the power and control that came with it. Her overseeing of the whole convent would, without a doubt, have included other mentally ill people as well. In fact, we know that she was not the only person holding some power in the Church to have had problems with mental illness, as not only chronicles but sometimes entries into the Calendar of Patent Rolls illustrate, such as one from the thirteenth century, recording a '[m]andate to the bishop and to Walter and John, archdeacons of Exeter, on the complaint of Peter, a deacon, to restore to him his prebend and other benefices in the diocese of Salisbury on recovery from his madness, caused by the loss of them, and injuries inflicted by the abbot of Reading and others'. That this could happen, and a 'mad' man won a case against the Church shows a stark contrast with the prejudice and the excesses inflicted by the same Church during the time of the Spanish Inquisition, only a few centuries later.

It could be argued, of course — and has, in fact, sometimes been argued[493] — that Hildegard's kind, respectful treatment did not happen in spite of her mental illness but because, as can be seen in several other cases of the time, it was not actually seen as a real mental illness. However, there are two facts that speak against this: first, that she herself was not even certain of it, that she struggled with it and that there were people who were so opposed to her explicitly due to her hearing voices they were ready to even get the Pope himself, the highest religious authority during the Middle Ages, involved to prevent her from becoming abbess. Secondly, according to Hildegard herself, hearing voices was not the only sign of her mental illness, though she herself did not put it in such words.[494]

Hallucinations, along with hearing voices, is another symptom that signals to modern readers that someone is suffering from a mental illness, though again, it was not seen as narrowly at the time and in some cases it was seen as a sign of a heavenly visitation, of having premonitions or being pious enough to be visited by saints. This did not always happen, though, or perhaps even very frequently, with auditory hallucinations being the exception. If hallucinations could not be immediately connected with a possible divine or devilish plan, it seems that often they were seen in the same way that we would view them today: as a sign of mental illness, or, as it would have been classified in Hildegard von Bingen's time, a sign of a diseased mind. This was at the very least something Hildegard herself feared, as she struggled with it and hoped that it was in fact a good sign, a sign of her piety, while being afraid it was the opposite.[495] Clearly, it was nowhere near as clear cut as it often seems nowadays, reading such beliefs purely theoretically, it seems it was never the fact that all people were convinced such voices or hallucinations came from God, or else from the devil or a diseased mind. There could be several different conclusions made about a single case, which shows that the system which included mental illnesses as part of possible human frailties was not at all static and did include margins for doubt, uncertainty or a change of mind.

The very fact that even for the sufferer themselves there could be no certainty would have made struggling with it all the more difficult, a difficulty that is no longer known to those afflicted with mental illness today. While it is still difficult and stigmatised, there is no fear that it might be the devil leading someone astray, no uncertainty as to whether the symptoms are actually a sign of something good or a sign of illness.[496]

That Hildegard managed to do all she did regardless is quite remarkable. It shows that she managed to succeed against all odds, against her own doubts, against the stigma of her mental illness, and the difficulty given by this illness itself. It also shows that she was given the space and the support to do it, even by the Pope. Since there is actually an indication that no money was offered to the Pope for this decision,[497] one way or another, this means that he probably came to the decision himself, deciding what he either believed or considered best for the Church. That not demoting a mentally ill woman was his decision shows that at least at the time, while there may have been stigma, it was nowhere near as pervasive as could be believed.

There is another interesting point that is brought up by Hildegard's case. She is very famous for her cures for her illness, and perhaps by observation of her own illness and her own state, she came to the conclusion that treating your body well, rather than subjecting it to gruesome treatments, also helped heal the mind.[498] Though some of her treatments are still rather foreign to us, some of her natural remedies are very close to the chemical ones used today.

Explicitly because of Hildegard's medical knowledge and the fact she managed to rise despite all odds, she is often regarded as being ahead of her time today, as a light in the supposed darkness of the Middle Ages.[499] This, however, ignores the fact that her ideas were brought on by observing herself and her surroundings, and that she received a lot of support too, support from people including the Pope himself. She seems to have been extraordinary in many ways, but her story was not impossible in the Middle Ages, nor is she somehow separated from the mediaeval times she lived in.

Though Hildegard struggled, she managed to not only achieve what she aimed for, to have a very productive life and help many others, she was also not bitter towards anyone and didn't consider anyone to be inferior. We are lucky to have many of her own words, and it is clear that she did not consider the society she lived in helplessly backwards, or herself a fish out of water due to her better understanding. On the contrary, while she did have criticisms of her surroundings, she was very fond of the world in general, and her greatest wish appears to have been to fit in.[500] This hardly suggests that she was so different from everyone that she should be considered a bright light in a dark world, an unusual occurrence that bordered on an impossibility because of the general backwardness, nastiness and meanness of those around her, and the lack of knowledge she was supposedly surrounded by.

This is not to say that she was not exceptional. She most definitely was and especially with some of her medicinal ideas, she was most definitely groundbreaking.[501] She was also contemporarily recognised as such, with some people even saying that it was this, not actually her mental illness, which turned several people against her and made them appeal to the Pope. A case of simple jealousy.[502] Not jealousy because she was so much smarter, to an unheard-of extent, but because her intelligence and her theories, especially her ability to heal illnesses, were admired so much that she had a lot of what today we would call 'fans'. Many of her enemies considered it to be ill-fitting, and perhaps some simply wished to be in her place.

Interestingly, this means that Hildegard was exactly the type of woman who is stereotypically claimed by many modern books to have been considered a witch and persecuted by the Church. It is by now long since known that Hildegard lived too early for witch hunts, which only happened several centuries after her death, and long before the Spanish Inquisition started as well. Even so, the claim of the Church being against smart women and wishing to keep them in ignorance has sadly proved very pervasive. Hildegard shows this was not the case — despite her mental illness, she could learn and teach and the Pope thought highly enough of her that he backed her in her a position of power and did not side with her enemies. This is very telling, both about the treatment of women at the time, and, more importantly for this book, about how mental illnesses were perceived and treated.

The last interesting aspect of Hildegard's case is that she was obviously able to work both through her doubts and the effects of her illness, which surely would have included more symptoms than just these two obvious ones of hearing voices and hallucinations. The excessive self-doubts she is known to have expressed as feelings might have been triggered by her mental illness, or been part of the mental illness, as might other ailments she is known to have had. Whether or not they were, if they were, how they were connected, and to which illness they point, is something that has been widely discussed in literature about her and about mediaeval culture in general and mediaeval religious culture in particular.[503] In fact, there is even a school of thought that she was not actually mentally ill at all, but that her visions were caused by a physical illness, such as migraines, which we know she suffered from. If this is at all possible, it is not for this book to discuss, but it definitely shows that even today, in some ways, we cannot analyse mental illnesses, or at least symptoms thereof, much better than our mediaeval forebears could. Hildegard's case does show that in some ways, while she did not consider herself cured, and while those who knew her well also knew she continued suffering, there was at least some treatment available to make the symptoms lessen, to make herself feel better.[504]

Hildegard was responsible for many breakthroughs in medicine, and continued being famous for it, with her recipes used throughout the Middle Ages,[505] and in fact, she was particularly popular in England. Though the fact she had heard voices and seen visions was widely known at the time and in later centuries, it was in no way used against her. On the contrary, despite the fact that the position of her enemies on this was a matter of public record, there is no indication that anyone ever took this stand after her death. Not long after her death she was awarded a sainthood as a smart and extraordinarily pious woman, perhaps showing one of the most impressive rises for a mediaeval woman, and also showcasing how life in the Church could actively help someone who suffered from a mental illness, or at the very least the symptoms thereof. It also shows that a mental illness was not the end of all hopes of achievement in life, not even if such an illness was suffered by a commoner, someone considered fairly insignificant at first.

Hildegard is still so famous today, alongside her musings about life, her struggles and even her recipes, because she wrote about them, and her books were famous even in the Middle Ages. Details of her struggles, and her life story in general, have been left to us, although, as with most except the most high-born, there are gaps in it which are hard to fill. This has not stopped historians and sometimes even fiction writers from trying to fill the gaps, whilst trying to find a trigger for her mental illnesses.[506] Naturally, this is something that, unless new evidence is found, can never truly be known. Interestingly, working with mental illness in fiction is something that was already being done in the Middle Ages and was a quite popular plot device.

Mental illness in mediaeval literature is a far more widespread subject than might be considered at first glance, and it is a subject that appears in many guises, in all sorts of texts. Most importantly, there are medical texts which would have been the most influential for people at the time, particularly those who did actually suffer from a mental illness.[507] This is the sort of book Hildegard von Bingen wrote, and it is immensely helpful for understanding what mediaeval people thought about mental illness, what different views there were and what treatments were used, which is why I have used it as a resource for Chapters 2 and 3. However, Hildegard's book is very dry and it is, in modern terms, non-fiction. While it therefore reflects mediaeval reality very nicely, it does not reflect what part mental illness played in stories of the Middle Ages, in what way it was incorporated in the very fabric of society, the way that fiction can.

Chapter 5

Mental health and mental illness in mediaeval literature

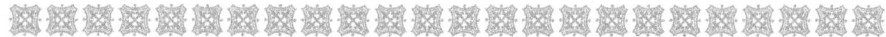

At the time, there were no novels as we know them today, which makes the search for fiction somewhat more difficult. What mediaeval fiction we have is in some ways much less coherent than we expect of fiction today. It has often been pieced together, consisting of different stories that appealed to the author, changed to reflect his tastes, his understanding of the world, of society and the issues it touches on. Today, such stealing would be called plagiarism, but this was not yet a concept at the time. This means that there is not always a certainty where a famous story came from, how many times it had been changed and how authentic the story was in its earliest form. Even so, due to the many changes usually made by an author when adapting the story to what he or she knew or wanted to convey, there is usually at least some chance for a historian, even one who does not know the origins of the original story, to make some deductions about the views of the author in question, as well as the views of society around the author, for whom the stories were usually written, or changed from their original form.

The most famous pieces of mediaeval literature, at least in the English-speaking world, must surely be *Le Morte D'Arthur*, a fifteenth-century retelling of the Arthurian legends by Thomas Malory, and *The Canterbury Tales*, written in the late-fourteenth century by Geoffrey Chaucer. Both books have very interesting insights into how mental illnesses were seen at the time.

In one of the most famous stories featured in *The Canterbury Tales*, 'The Miller's Tale', madness plays a significant role. However, in this story it is only a pretence of madness, something that is used by one character to dupe another. The person being duped, a 'simple' carpenter, is portrayed as very simple-minded and therefore easy to trick, but there is no suggestion in the story that the symptoms feigned by the more clever character, the one who is duping the carpenter, are in any way meant to be exaggerated, wrong, or something that should have been easy to spot as a ruse by a more clever man.[508]

In the context of the story, the madness is feigned by a scholar lodging with a carpenter and his much younger wife. The carpenter loves his wife but is very jealous and afraid of her cheating on him, which is exactly what she intends to do, egged on by the scholar who wishes to sleep with her. However, because the carpenter is very attentive to his wife and said to be 'guarding her closely', the two would-be lovers have to hatch a plan. Eventually, the scholar decides on pretending to be mad, to eventually convince the carpenter that he has found out that another flood like Noah's flood was coming.

The description of how this scholar [Nicholas] pretends to be mad are very interesting, as shown in the text: 'And there sat Nicholas, still as a stone, and kept on gaping up into the air'.[509] His host, the carpenter, reacts thusly:

> 'On hearing this the carpenter began to cross himself and "Help us, St Frideswide!" He said "No man can tell what may betide. He's fallen in a fit or some insanity, and all because of all this astroboly. As all along I thought that it would be.
>
> One shouldn't pry into God's mystery. Yes, the unlettered man is blessed indeed Who doesn't know a thing except his Creed! Much the same fate befell, it seems to me, That other student of astroboly: He walked the fields stargazing, to foresee What might befall; and suddenly fell in A claypit — something that he'd not foreseen. But all the same, I swear by St Thomas I'm most upset about Fly Nicholas. He shall be scolded for his studying If I've got anything to do with it — Yes, that he shall, by Jesus, heaven's King!"'[510]
>
> And there sat Nicholas, still as a stone, And kept on gaping up into the air. The carpenter, thinking he was in

a fit, Took Nicholas by the shoulders, gripped them tight And shook him hard, and yelled with all his might: "What, Nicholas! What! Look down for God's sake! Think on Christ's suffering! Awake, awake! The sign of the cross defend you from all harm, From sprites and elves!".'[511]

It is interesting that the clearest indicator of Nicholas's supposed madness is what could best be described, in modern terms, as catatonia, the exact same symptoms Henry VI would have when his mental illness first showed itself in 1453, nearly a century after *The Canterbury Tales* were written. The reaction the carpenter has to this is also telling, as it is meant to be seen as stupid and wrong. Though it might have been the first instinct to shake someone who did not react, it was not seen as the smart and most promising cause of action. This is presented as something that everyone should know; that the carpenter is in the wrong for not knowing. This is particularly interesting since that sort of illness is hardly all that widespread and chances would be that not only Geoffrey Chaucer himself had never seen it, but nor would most commoners have had. This suggests that there was at least some knowledge even about obscure mental illnesses around at the time, even if it was only by applying common sense to situations that might arise when dealing with mental illness and people suffering from it.

The story goes on by saying that upon being 'awoken' from his madness, the scholar tells the carpenter he has found out that there will be another flood like the Deluge, something he manages to convince the carpenter with. The handyman makes preparations for this supposed next Deluge, believing blindly in everything the scholar tells him, down to the exact date. When this date comes, he hides in a bathtub so he can float on the water, leaving his wife unsupervised and able to sleep with the scholar.

Through a weird and deliberately unrealistic chain reaction, he eventually comes to believe that the Deluge is actually happening when hearing the scholar call for water, and cuts loose his bathtub to float, causing him to simply crash through the roof and looking like a complete fool, or rather, as the text puts it:

> '[...] when he spoke, he was at once borne down By both Fly Nicholas and Alison. For they told everybody he was mad, So frightened of a fancied "Nowell's Flood" That

in his folly he had gone and bought Three kneading-tubs, and hung them from the roof, And that he had then begged them, for God's love, To sit with him to keep him company. Folk began laughing at his lunacy; Up at the roof they peered and stared and gaped, And treated his misfortune as a joke. No matter what the carpenter might say, It was no use, none took him seriously. Their sworn testimony so beat him down, He was reputed mad by the whole town, For all the scholars sided with the other, Saying "The man's a crackpot, my dear fellow".

So that the whole affair became a joke.'[512]

Interestingly, the text ends with everyone thinking him mad, not the scholar, with the narrative agreeing on it at least somewhat. For modern readers, this is obvious; for mediaeval readers, this would have been as obvious, if for different reasons. One sign of the carpenter's madness is constantly referring to his faith in God and his beliefs, yet not even being aware of the most basic tenets of this belief system he puts all his trust in. The mere fact that he believes that a second Deluge is going to happen marks him as not only a stupid man but one who is not aware of the teachings of the Bible, which explicitly says God Himself promised that this would never happen again.[513]

This very fact, the neglect to believe in God's own words and God's mercy, marks the carpenter as rather mad to Chaucer's contemporary audience, but there is another, rather interesting, aspect of fourteenth-century understanding of madness inherent in the portrayal of this character. Nicholas, the scholar, is shown to be a very intelligent and highly educated man, who is able, with his knowledge and education, to manipulate someone, though his ruse is done in such a way that it would only fool someone who is himself not very smart. The carpenter, on the other hand, is portrayed not only as ill-educated, which is not in itself portrayed as in any way bad or regrettable, but also as actively scorning education. In fact, when Nicholas plays mad, he explicitly says that he believes that too much education, and a preoccupation with knowing too much, leads to madness:

'"Help us, St Frideswide!" He said "No man can tell what may betide. He's fallen in a fit or some insanity, and all because of all this astroboly. As all along I thought that it would be. One shouldn't pry into God's mystery. Yes, the unlettered man is blessed indeed. Who doesn't know a thing except his Creed!".'[514]

This is, in itself, only the statement of someone in a story inside a story. To make any judgements from this to the opinion of the author would be a ridiculous stretch. However, the story is structured in such a way as to not only prove the carpenter holding this opinion wrong, but to actively portray him as 'mad', or mentally ill. A part of this, of course, is due to him saying he only has his belief and it drives a man crazy, into mental illness, to have any more knowledge than that, only to prove that he does not even, in fact, have the beliefs. His beliefs are so uneducated, he is so unknowledgeable about these beliefs, that he can easily be convinced, by someone he considers a madman at that, that something that is diametrically opposed to these beliefs is about to happen. He does, in short, not have his beliefs, just a loose set of uninformed ideas about the religion he considers his only need in life.

Being uneducated about such basic tenets of Christianity was unforgivable for a Christian at the time, and the character was obviously set up to be mocked for this. However, the very fact that the character who considers too much knowledge to lead to madness is later himself shown as mad, mad in fact explicitly due to having too little knowledge, his reliance on faith backfiring because of him placing so much reliance on it that he failed to even understand important parts of it, is certainly telling as to the understanding of madness at the time this story was written.

Moreover, the fact that the narrative itself points out that he is not only unaware of such religious fine points but also of some basic facts of life, the most important for the story being not to marry someone either out of his league, much older or much younger. The whole premise of the story is based on him ignoring that, and while such marriages were hardly unusual, such a statement so early in the story does serve to mark the carpenter out as at best silly, at worst somewhat mad in expecting it to work.

There is also the fact that he is shown as being ready to believe what his houseguests says, shortly after him waking up from what the carpenter believes to have been a spell of madness. This notion of it being important to listen to what a madman, or someone who recently showed signs of madness, says, is in itself treated as a sign of madness on the carpenter's part.

Seeing as it is only a story within a story, it is possible to place too much reliance on the picture of mental illness presented in the story, and as such, to make conclusions from it that could very easily be faulty. However, even so, it is clear that to make a story be actually interesting to an audience, there has to be something the readers or listeners can identify with. There is no evidence Geoffrey Chaucer wanted to have a different value system in his stories, even the stories within the story, to present a point of view that not only was not shared by his listeners and readers but was not understood. The former would have been perfectly doable, and in fact, some of the stories told in *The Canterbury Tales* actively rely on it. The latter would not only have made no sense for fourteenth-century audiences but would make just as little sense today; after all, to interest people in a story, the narrative needs to offer something with which the readers can identify, even if said identification is later subverted by the author.

Therefore, there can be a discussion as to why and how the presentation of 'madness' in 'The Miller's Tale' has to be some sort of reflection to what was said, thought and believed about mental illness at the time of writing the story. This means that, however one reads it, as either in sync with the morals the story itself passes on or as mocking them, a correlation between learning and mental illness was thought to exist, a theory that is also found elsewhere. This has been discussed in Chapter 2.3, though it is presented rather colourfully in this tale. A theory we know existed at some point during the Middle Ages was that the theory endorsed by the carpenter — that of trying too hard to understand the world as made by God without leaving any place for miracles — did indeed drive someone into mental illness. That there was also an idea as to the opposite, of not only lack of education but scorn of education, complete reliance on God alone without also trusting the ingenuity of men, and that this could also lead to mental illness, is not a theory that we know existed at the time, though such a thing is hard to categorically say. It is all but impossible for any theory to not have existed at some point, but if this one did, it was a rather obscure one, which was not written down anywhere that has survived the centuries and was not one that was much in discourse.

It could very well be that this in itself was a judgement of the author on his character of the miller, who was telling this tale in the context of the story. Perhaps, it was his own opinion, but veiled in such a way. There is absolutely no way of saying.

It is usually assumed by Chaucer scholars that the story is meant to spoof both those who rely too much on human knowledge without factoring in God, or perverting the word of God for their own means, as well as those who blindly believe anything about religion they are told, without asking any questions or even informing themselves about what they were meant to be guided by and have based their entire life philosophy on.[515] If so, it would mean that the author considered both these extremes to be madness.

There is, however, something of a tendency in literary criticism, especially for works as famous as *The Canterbury Tales*, to see the opinion of the person writing the criticism reflected in their reading of the story. It is especially possible in this case, since the understanding of madness and mental illness in the tale, and its reflection on society, has changed as understanding of these issues changed over time. As such, the story was considered to be indicative of supposedly backwards mediaeval ideas of mental illness during the Enlightenment,[516] with the carpenter intended to be the most sympathetic character.[517] However, during the Renaissance, the scholar Nicholas was considered the most sympathetic character, as he rejected what was seen as mediaeval understanding of religion as represented by the carpenter.[518] Only in recent years has the theory of there being a middle way, and this middle way being the one intended by Geoffrey Chaucer, really started to take hold.[519] Therefore, it would be somewhat conceited to say that any one view was intended by the author, particularly as there is no real way of knowing his intentions. All that can be said with some certainty is that there is some rather curious reflection of knowledge, lack thereof and its influence on mental illness. Even if it was a spoof, or a complete reversal, of something that was believed at the time, a connection was there — of too much knowledge, or too little knowledge and blind reliance on faith, which not only led to madness but was considered a form of madness it in itself. This sounds like a rather radical concept, especially for a time stereotyped as being almost exclusively shaped by a mindset such as the fictional carpenter shows. At the very least, what can be said is that this sort of mindset was not only not expected, but mocking it in a fictional context, if perhaps not in a work of scholarship, was considered perfectly acceptable. Moreover, mocking someone who exhibited such a mindset in a fictional context as mentally ill and portraying them as a laughing stock was not only considered acceptable, but perfectly fine entertainment for the masses, something that had no repercussions of any sort. It is, therefore, another sign that the Middle Ages were nowhere near as backwards as is often claimed, even if it is not too telling as to what was really thought about mental health, mental illness and its connection with knowledge, learning, the lack thereof and blind faith. All that can be said with certainty is that there was considered to be a connection of some sort, for the story to make sense for the audience it was created for.

A similar dilemma is posed by the other most famous piece of late mediaeval English literature: *Le Morte D'Arthur*, written in the mid-fifteenth century by Thomas Malory.[520] As a retelling of the Arthurian legends which were very famous at the time and in the centuries before, we do not have the same problem that we do with many mediaeval works of literature, of not knowing where the stories came from, though *Le Morte D'Arthur* is the first work of these legends that puts them all together. It appears to have been a very famous and very popular work, with some parts of it being among the first books printed in England and being found in the possession of at least one king — Richard III — and one queen consort — Richard's niece, Elizabeth of York.[521] The stories as penned and interpreted by Malory resonated with all echelons of society, which makes looking at what they say about society, and, in this case, specifically about mental illnesses and madness, particularly interesting.

There are two parts explicitly dealing with what is called 'madness' within the text. The first is probably the more famous one for modern audiences, who may have read the same stories in many different variations several times before, including in adaptations for television and in other media: the story of Lancelot, King Arthur's right-hand man.

In fact, the 'love story' of Lancelot and Elaine is rather problematic for modern readers, and Malory's narrative, though often a bit disjointed, makes this very clear from the first. Very famously, Lancelot is portrayed as in love with his queen, King Arthur's wife, Queen Guinivere. This has a lot of potential for conflict in any story, of course, and it is milked for just that conflict in Malory's book. Perhaps, the twist he added was more surprising to mediaeval readers than it is for modern readers who already know the story well before reading Malory's version. Lancelot wishes Guinevere would have an affair with him, which she does not want. However, there is a lady called Elaine who is in love with Lancelot and wants to have an affair with him, but he rejects her. Knowing he has eyes only for Guinevere, Elaine takes a potion that makes her look like Guinevere and pretends to seduce him. Lancelot, thinking she is actually the woman he loves, sleeps with her.[522]

By modern standards, this is rape by deception and Lancelot is a rape victim. This is never spelled out in the book, nor does the deception, in itself, appear to be a problem for either the narrative or the author, who used such a device more than once, even in the very beginning of the book, a deception of the same sort leading to King Arthur's conception in the first place. This is never shown as in any way a bad thing, and there is no allusion made to the fact that this is rape, though even by mediaeval standards it would be.

However, the book is concerned with the fallout of such actions. In the case of King Arthur's mother, she finds out that she is pregnant and that, purely logically, her husband can't be the father, as he was in a battle in which he died at the time the conception took place. She remarried, whilst pregnant, and is said to be ecstatic at finding out that she married the father of her baby and is not actually pretending to him to be carrying his baby. This is not exactly overly plausible, but it does solve a fictional situation neatly, which is then never mentioned from then on.[523]

Such a neat solution does not happen for Lancelot, who, upon sleeping with Elaine in disguise, finds himself in a relationship with her, a relationship he does not want and feels trapped in. This is something that eventually causes his mental illness. The very knowledge of having slept with Elaine, whom he does not want to sleep with, rather than Guinevere, sends him somewhat mad, a situation that causes several other characters, including King Arthur himself, to speculate that he is love mad, driven slightly crazy with the emotion he is assumed to feel for Elaine. This is not true and known by the reader to not be true, and there is a quite plausible section of the book in which Lancelot struggles mentally with having been, in modern terms, raped, hoodwinked into a relationship with his rapist and then assumed to be actually deeply in love with her. Added to that, in a problem that the narrative shows as something that is attacking his mental health, is that he is in love with someone else, and cannot tell his best friend, King Arthur, nor any of his other friends about it, nor about the way he was hoodwinked by Elaine in the first place. Because telling them would be admitting that he was ready to betray King Arthur and very happy to sleep with whom he assumed was his wife.

Lancelot's reactions to all this are portrayed as more and more erratic, and are meant to be that. He jumps from his bedroom window in his nightshirt, not caring that he is getting stung by thorns upon finding out he slept with Elaine, not Guinevere. He acts strangely towards King Arthur and everyone else at King Arthur's court, and eventually, he leaves the court entirely to fight adventures in some other part of the world, not returning to court for several years.[524]

Interestingly, all this is presented in the narrative as 'mad' — mentally ill, in modern terms — and this madness is described as having been brought on by the strain of these extreme situations surrounding Lancelot's love and sex life, and by not being able to share these situations with anyone. This would be considered to be emotionally stressful in the modern day as well, to such a point that some sort of mental illness in reaction would hardly be considered unusual.

Lancelot's pain is portrayed vividly. The reader sees him react to the stress and the pain of being raped. They also see him deal with having nobody to turn to, and being hoodwinked and forced into a relationship with his rapist. Added to that, his friends are portrayed as believing he is happy in this relationship and in love with his rapist. The portrayal of his reaction to this and the psychological damage inflicted by this is perhaps the most realistic part of the whole of *Le Morte D'Arthur*. It is a book otherwise filled not only with magic, potions and other magical plot devices, but also not exactly featuring the most plausible of characters and character reactions.

Of course, what sort of book this tale comes from has to be taken into account before making any conclusions on what the presentation of mental illness in Lancelot means for the understanding of the intended audience of these issues. After all, the book in itself is not entirely meant to be taken seriously, even assuming that the audience believed the Arthurian legends on which it was based. Too obviously there are clear problems with reality and logic, which are obviously meant to be noticed. This is not the only Arthurian legend to deal with the source material this way; there is a modern-day novel, called *The Once and*

Future King, written by T. H. White, which does the exact same thing, playing with explicit and deliberate anachronisms to sell the point of several of these stories,[525] which is exactly what Malory does as well.

However, it is harder to work out just which parts of Malory's book are meant to be such deliberate inaccuracies, things his audience would obviously recognise as being deliberately wrong, and what is not. After all, it is known that in the fifteenth century, there was still a very widespread belief in things such as magic, and with nowhere near the stigma these beliefs would have later. It also seems like the Arthurian legends themselves were considered to be true in essence, with King Arthur, Lancelot and all the other famous characters being real historical people.[526]

Therefore, there are two problems when analysing the story for signs of how Thomas Malory himself understood mental illness and its effects, and how it was understood in the fifteenth century in general. Again, it has to be pointed out that a story could not have been reasonably told, and much less have resonated with such a large and widespread audience, if it included values and understanding of issues that were unknown to the intended audience. It could, however, have carried some of these values and judgement of issues over from previous retellings, and therefore have made sense to an audience who actually knew the stories before, even if they contained different world views from the ones that were held by the audience in the fifteenth century.

It is important to say that it was the common practice for authors adapting stories in the Middle Ages, to change them in such a way as to fit perhaps not their own views but those of his or her intended audience, or at the very least, change them in such a way that the audience would be able to understand and be able to judge the values exhibited by characters in a story, or even by the narrative itself, and there is evidence of Malory doing just that. To what extent is hard to say, and literary critics have had different opinions of this for a long time. Some of them consider it to be only marginally changed from original legends, while others consider the changes to be very strong, and even see an allegory in some of the stories for not only several events in the author's life but also for some of the upheaval in the country that happened when he was writing the book, the series of conflicts known to history as the Wars of the Roses.

Whether or not this is true is of no concern to this book, with it only being significant to see that literary critics agree on there being a connection to Malory's own views, or at least the views he found himself surrounded by in his life. As such, it is a fair assumption that he portrayed Lancelot's own descent into madness in a way that would be understandable to him and his intended audience.

This would indicate once more that there was a strong understanding between mental illness and very traumatic events, a connection that gives us more evidence as to what was understood during the Middle Ages, evidence which has been discussed above in Chapter 2.3. What is most interesting, though, is that in Lancelot's story, there is an indication that such traumatic events could in fact also be of sexual nature, and rape by deception being considered to be just as likely to trigger a descent into mental illness. Naturally, with this happening twice in the book, and once being dismissed, Malory does not exactly make a strong case for this, but in Lancelot's case, he is very explicit about it. The scene in which he describes Lancelot's reaction to finding out he has been hoodwinked, being made to sleep with someone he has no interest in sleeping with, is tough to read and gives a good insight into the way that traumatic events could affect someone's mental health.

As with most fiction written at the time, the book is full of complete exaggerations of the characters' behaviour, but such instances are usually marked by the language used. This does not happen in this case and is intended to show an actual breakdown by Lancelot. As such, it can very well be argued that there was an underlying understanding of such sexually aggressive behaviour causing mental illnesses in the victim. Certainly, it is meant to be very sympathetic, and as such, it must have been something that Malory and his audience could understand and sympathise with, not a reaction they would not understand or even find silly and over the top.

The same also counts for Lancelot's reaction, him slipping increasingly into 'madness', as the whole situation unfolds. It is over the top and none of the symptoms he exhibits really have a real-life counterpart. However, what it meant to show is very obvious, and as such it is an interesting case of mental illness treated in a very sympathetic, if rather exaggerated way, and it being considered a natural reaction to traumatic events.[527]

That Lancelot is, and remains throughout the story, a very sympathetic character is equally rather telling. This is not the case in Geoffrey Chaucer's 'The Miller's Tale', in which the carpenter who is thought to be mad becomes a laughing stock both inside the story and for the audience. Lancelot, however, is a victim of circumstances and his mental illness considered both within the story as a sad reaction to someone else's crime against him, and the circumstances where he finds himself innocent; and it is presented like this in the narrative as well, with the obvious intention to make the readers sympathise with him and root for a happy ending.

Lancelot, though the most famous example, is not the only character in *Le Morte D'Arthur* to be stricken with madness due to love gone awry. Another sympathetic character, Lamorak, is as well, though in his case it is simply being unable to be with the woman he loves, and is not as extreme as Lancelot's reaction to the rather more traumatic situations his character goes through in the story.[528] However, what can be seen from this is that strong negative emotions, such as being unable to be with your lover, or even worse being raped, hoodwinked and forced into a relationship, are portrayed as very natural triggers for mental illness with these resulting mental illnesses treated very sympathetically. That Malory chose very sympathetic characters as the ones who suffered from mental illness does not have to have been his decision; instead, he would have simply continued a tradition from the legends he was adapting. However, his decision to portray them so very sympathetically while suffering from mental illness, and the illnesses so graphically, must have been his decision and is very telling. Obviously, he felt that it was easy to pack a punch and make his audience sympathise with these characters like this, rather than thinking it would repulse them and make them scorn these characters.

Naturally, looking at these two most famous examples of late mediaeval English literature is hardly a comprehensive study of the depiction of mental illness in mediaeval fiction, but it is certainly a start, and it shows that different views of mental illness and those afflicted with it were as present in fiction as they were in real life, and the characters which are portrayed with mental illness are just as varied as the people stricken with mental illness in real life are. Clearly then, allowing for literary exaggeration, mental illness in fiction was used to mirror these issues in real life.

In conclusion, we can say that like today, mental illnesses were considered a very complex subject, with different cultures at different times having different ideas about it, about where it came from, what constituted a mental illness, how it should be treated and what people afflicted by it were like. It was not automatically considered stigmatising and in fact, was treated with much more compassion than we today associate with the Middle Ages.

Appendices

1. *Ingulph's Chronicle of the Abbey of Croyland* on John Beaufort, Duke of Somerset:

While these years were rolling onward in their headlong flight, the lady Margaret, duchess of Clarence, died, and John, Earl of Somerset, her son and heir, who had passed fifteen years in captivity with the French, was ransomed for an immense sum of money, and so returned to England. Upon this, among other matters, he took possession of the manor of Depyng, and whole multitudes of the district flocked forth to meet him, each one endeavouring to be avenged upon his neighbour, and thinking himself fortunate in being enrolled among the number of his servants. The people of Depyng were especially elated, as though a prophet had risen among them; escorting him about on every side, promising great things, and suggesting still more; while by the voice of a herald they proclaimed him lord of the whole march.

Upon this, his heart was elevated to a lofty pitch, and, being puffed up by the great applause of the populace, his horn was exalted too greatly on high. Forthwith, tolls were levied by his servants in the vills; and the cattle of all were driven away from the marches and, when driven as far as Depyng, detained; nor were they allowed to be redeemed without a payment and acknowledgment of him as lord of the demesne. In his name the embankment between Kenulphston and Croyland was raised anew, and all transit and leading of necessaries from his manors through those parts entirely forbidden to the abbat. Upon this; the abbat by bill complained to the king of the injury done to him, whereby the earl's wrath was still more inflamed. Threats too were daily spread abroad against his monks and servants, nor did any one dare venture to go that way for the purpose of transacting business. At length, by act of Parliament, from an earl he was created a duke, and, God so ordaining it, was sent upon an expedition [sic] in parts beyond the sea. In the meantime, however, the venerable father, abbat John, fearing lest in his absence his servants might still further run riot against him by committing injuries, hastened for the purpose of holding a conference with him, to a distant quarter of England, in the most sultry season of the year, and in a summer remarkable for its heat, the said duke being then at his castle at Corfe, with the intention of immediately crossing over. Here too he had to submit to considerable delays, being under frequent apprehensions of attempts being made by the servants on his life; but at last, after earnestly beseeching his favour, he obtained letters directed to the duke's seneschal in these parts, ordering that the whole matters in dispute should stand over until his return, and that in the meantime no opportunity should be taken of inflicting injury on the said abbat and his servants.

The business on which he had crossed over being settled in a short time, the duke returned amid much pomp to England; but being accused of treason there, was forbidden to appear in the king's presence. The noble heart of a man of such high rank upon his hearing this most unhappy news, was moved to extreme indignation; and being unable to bear the stain of so great a disgrace, he accelerated his death by putting an end to his existence, it is generally said: prefering thus to cut short his sorrow, rather than pass a life of misery, labouring under so disgraceful a charge.

2. On the first rebellion of the Duke of York, 1455, and the failure to use his insanity as a justification:

Copy of part of a letter written from Bruges to the Archbishop of Ravenna.
We left London on the 27th May and at that time there was nothing new; my lord of Somerset ruled as usual. Subsequently I learned here yesterday, by letters which came straight from Sandwich to Dunkirk, that fresh disturbances broke out in England a few days after my

departure. A great part of the nobles have been in conflict, and the Duke of Somerset, the Earl of Northumberland and my lord of Clifford are slain, with many other lords and knights on both sides. The Duke of Somerset's son, who presented the collars of the king, was mortally wounded; my lord of Buckingham and his son are hurt. The Duke of York has done this, with his followers. On the 24th he entered London and made a solemn procession to St. Pauls. They say he has demanded pardon from the king for himself and his men, and will have it. He will take up the government again, and some think that the affairs of that kingdom will now take a turn for the better. If that be the case, we can put up with this inconvenience. No one comes from Calais as the passages are guarded. We should hear further particulars from merchants, messengers and those who come. I send your lordship these particulars, as you will be glad to hear them even though the news seems unpleasant.

Bruges, the last day of May, 1455.
Postscript on the 3rd of June. — I have further news of the battle in England brought by one who came here from Calais. They say that on the 21st of May the king left Westminster with many lords, including the Duke of Somerset, to hold a council at Leicester (a le cestre), eight miles (sic) from London. They went armed because they suspected that the Duke of York would also go there with men at arms. That day they travelled twenty miles to the abbey of St. Albans. On the 22nd the king set out to continue his journey, but when they were outside the town they were immediately attacked by York's men, and many perished on both sides. The Duke of Somerset was taken and forthwith beheaded. With his death the battle ceased at once and, without loss of time, the Duke of York went to kneel before the king and ask pardon for himself and his followers, as they had not done this in order to inflict any hurt upon his Majesty, but in order to have Somerset. Accordingly the king pardoned them, and on the 23rd the king and York and all returned to London. On the 24th they made the solemn procession, and now peace reigns. The king has forbidden any one to speak about it upon pain of death (*il Re ha mandato Bando a pena di vita, non se ne parli*). The Duke of York has the government, and the people are very pleased at this (*il duca de Jorlz ha il governo et li popoli se ne tengono molto contenti*).

3. *Whethamsted's Register*, speaking about Henry VI and his mental illness:

A disease and disorder of such a sort overcame the king that he lost his wits and memory for a time, and nearly all his body was so uncoordinated and out of control that he could neither walk, nor hold his head upright, nor easily move from where he sat. [...] his mother's stupid offspring, not his father's, a son greatly degenerated from his father, who did not cultivate the art of war ... a mild spoken, pious king, but half-witted in affairs of state.

4. Richard, Duke of York, Richard, Earl of Warwick and Richard, Earl of Salisbury, speaking against Henry VI and his government, and their failure to use Henry's mental illness as a justification:

Most Crystyne kyng, ryghte hyghe and rayghtye Prince, and oure most drad souuerayne lorde, after as humble recommendacione to youre hyghe excellence as we suffice. Oure trewe entent to the prosperyte and augmentacione of youre hyghe estate, and to the commone wele of this reaume, hath be showd vn to youre hyghenesse in suche wrytyng as we made thereof. And ouer that, an endenture sygned by oure handes in the churche Cathedralle of Worcestre comprehendyng the preef of the trouthe and dewte that, God knowethe, we here to youre seyde estate and to the preemynence and prerogatif therof, we sent vn to youre good grace by the prior of the saide churche and diuerse other doctours, and among other, by master William Lynwode, dctour of diuinite, whyche myriistred vnto us seuerally the blessed Body of God our Lorde Jhesu; sacred whereoponne, we and euery of vs deposyd for oure sayde trouthe and dewtee accordyng to the tenure of the seyde endenture. And syth that tyme, we haue certyfyed at large in wrytyng and by mouthe by Garter kyng of Armes, nat only to youre sayde hyghenesse, but also to the good and worthy lordes beyng aboute youre moste noble presence, the largenesse of oure sayde trouthe and dewte, and oure entent and oure disposicione to seche alle the mocions that myghte serue conuenyently to thaffirmacione therof, and to oure parfyte suertees from suche inconuenient and unreuerent geopardyes, as we haue ben put ynne diuerse tymes herebefore. Wherof we haue cause to make, and owe to make, suche exclamacione and compleynt, nat withoute reasone, as ys nat unknowen to alle the sayd worthy lordes and to alle his lande, and wolle offre vs to youre hyghe presence to the same entent, yef we myghte so do wythe oure sayde sewrte, whiche onely causethe vs to kepe aboute vs suche felyshyp as we do in oure leeffulle. And hereto we haue forborne and avoyded alle thynges that myghte serue to the effusione of Crysten blood, of the drede that we haue of God and of youre royalle mageste; and haue also eschewed to approche your seyde moste noble presence, of the humble obeysaunce and reuerence whereon we haue and duryng oure lyfe wolle haue the same. And yet neuertheles, we here that we be proclamed and defamed in oure name vnryghtefully, vniawfully, and sauyng youre hyghe reuerence, vntrewly, and otherwyse, that God knowethe, then we haue yeue cause; knowyng certaynly that the blessed and noble entent of youre sayde goode grace and the ryghtwysnesse thereof ys, to take, repute, and accepte youre trew and lowly sugettys, and that it accordethe neyther with youre sayde entent, ne wythe youre wylle or pleasure, that we shuld be otherwyse take or reputed. And ouer that, oure lordshyppes and tenauntes bene of hyghe vyolence robbed and spoyled, ayenst youre peese and lawes and alle ryghtewysnesse. We therefore, as we suffice, beseche youre sayde good grace, to take, repute, and receyue thervnto oure sayde trouthe and entent, whiche to God ys know, as we shewe it by the seyde tenure of the sayde endenture, and nat apply youre sayde blessednesse ne the grete ryghtewysnesse and equite whereinne God hathe euer endowed youre hyghe nobeley, to thymportune impacience and violence of suche persones as entende of extreme malyce to precede vnder the shadow of youre hyghe myghte and presence to oure destruccione, for suche inordinate couetyse, whereof God ys nat pleased, as they haue to oure landes, offices, and goodes, not lettyng or sparyng therefore to put suche thyngys in alle lamentable and to sorowfulle geopardy, as moot in alle wyse take effect by the mystery of Goddys wille and power, nor nat hauyng regarde to theffusione of Crystyne blood, ne any tendrenesse to the noble blood of thys lond suche as serue to the tuicione and defens therof, ne nat weyng the losse of youre trew liegemenne of youre sayde reame, that God defende whiche knowethe oure entent, and that we haue avoyded therfro, as fer as we may with oure sewertees, nat of any drede that we haue of the sayde persones, but onely of the drede of God and of youre sayde hyghenesse, and nat wylle vse oure sayde defence vnto the tyme that we be provoked of necessyte, whereof we calle heuene and erthe in to wyttenesse and recorde; and therynne beseche God to be oure Juge, and to delyuer vs accordyng to oure sayde entent, and oure sayde trouthe and dutie to youre seyde hyghenesse, and to the sayde commone wele. Most Crysten Kyng, ryghte hyghe and myghtye Prince, and moste drad souerayne lorde, we beseche oure blessed Lord to preserue youre honoure and estate in ioye and felycite. Wretynne at Ludlow, the x. day of Octobre. R. York, R. Warrewyk, R. Salesbury

5. Excerpts from the Act of Parliament condemning Henry VI and his reign, 1461:

When this petition had been read, heard and fully understood in the aforesaid parliament, by the advice and assent of the lords spiritual and temporal and the commons of the realm of England being in the same parliament, and by authority of the same, it was answered in the following form: Let it be done as it is desired. Thirdly, at your coming to your said city, it pleased your noble and benign grace, of the abundant tenderness that it pleased you to bear in natural love towards your said subjects, regarding their defence and security with heartfelt and sympathetic affection, and their mournful complaints with gracious benevolence, to take upon you, to the pleasure of God and the infinite and assured joy of all your said subjects, the rule and governance of the said realm, to which you are rightfully and naturally entitled by birth; and with all reasonable haste to leave for the said northern regions, organising, arming and leading your troops, like a victorious prince, for the defence and salvation of your said realm and subjects, against your adversary Henry, late called King Henry VI, and his forces, not only your rebels, but also Scots and Frenchmen, your enemies, whom he incited and retained to assist him, equipped and armed, against your said majesty; who, not deterred by any danger, peril or risk, dedicating your most noble person in your knightly and princely courage to the said defence and salvation, met the said forces of your said adversary in your county of York, on Palm Sunday last, where battle was joined and engaged against your said magnificence. In which it pleased Almighty God to send you by his grace recovery of your right, and victory against your said adversary, enemies and rebels; whom the fear of your mighty power and of the renown of your knightly and princely prowess, drove and chased out of your said realm, without lingering, into Scotland.

And since in the time of the usurped reign of your said adversary Henry, late called King Henry VI, extortion, murder, rape, the shedding of innocent blood, riot and unrighteousness were commonly practised in your said realm without punishment; we are absolutely sure that it will please your said good grace to promote everything that may advance the said common weal, the exercise of justice and righteousness, and the punishment of the great and terrible offenders, extortioners and rioters, and to have pity, compassion and mercy upon the innocents, to God's pleasure; whom we beseech long to continue and prosper your noble reign over us, your true and lowly subjects, in honour, joy and felicity.

And that it be announced and judged, by the said advice, assent and authority, that the said Henry, late earl of Derby, for the said raising of war against the said King Richard, then his sovereign lord, and the violent capture, imprisonment, unjust usurpation, intrusion and terrible cruel murder of him, contrary to his faith and allegiance, wickedly and unrightfully offended and harmed the royal majesty of his said sovereign lord; and that the same Henry unrightfully, against the law, conscience and custom of the realm of England, usurped the said crown and lordship; and that he, and also Henry, late called King Henry V his son, and the said Henry, late called King Henry VI, the son of the said Henry, late called King Henry V, occupied the said realm of England and lordship of Ireland, and exercised its governance, by unrightful intrusion and usurpation, and in no other way; and that the taking of possession and entry into the exercise of the royal estate, dignity, reign and governance of the said realm of England and lordship of Ireland by our said sovereign liege lord King Edward IV, on the said 4 March; and the removal of the said Henry, late called King Henry VI, from the exercise, occupation, usurpation, intrusion, reign and governance of the same realm and lordship, done by our said sovereign and liege lord King Edward IV on the said 4 March, was and is rightful, lawful, and according to the laws and customs of the said realm, and so ought to be taken, held, considered and accepted.

And notwithstanding the foregoing, the said Henry, usurper, late called King Henry VI, continuing in his old rancour and malice, using fraud and malicious deceit and dissimulation contrary to truth and conscience, which does not sort with the honour of any Christian prince, with the intention that the said agreement, concord and act should not take proper effect and the matters and things described above be frustrated, that is to say, so that the said Duke Richard should not have or enjoy the same castles, manors, lands and tenements, name, title, reverence and worship described above, or his sons and heirs succeed to the said crowns, royal estate, dignity and lordship, according to the tenor, form and effect of the said agreement, concord and act, by all possible devious schemes and deceitful ways and means, intended and covertly urged, incited and instigated the final destruction, murder and death of the said Duke Richard and his sons, that is to say, of our said present sovereign lord King Edward IV, then earl of March, and of the noble Lord Edmund, earl of Rutland; and to bring about his damnable and malicious purpose, he encouraged, incited and stirred by writings and other messages the dukes of Exeter and Somerset and other lords being then in the northern regions of this realm. Whereupon, at Wakefield in the county of York, the said duke of Somerset falsely and traitorously, horribly, cruelly and tyrannously murdered the same noble prince, the duke of York, on Tuesday 30 December last; and also the worthy and good lords Edmund, earl of Rutland, brother of our said sovereign lord, and Richard, earl of Salisbury; and not content with this, they had them beheaded after they were dead with abominable cruelty and spite, out of their insatiable malice, contrary to all humanity and nobility.

6. The Act of Parliament reversing William Beaumont, Viscount Beaumont's attainder, November 1485:

To the king our sovereign lord; your true subject William Beaumont, knight, prays your highness most humbly that where by an act of parliament made in the parliament of Edward IV late king of England, held at Westminster on 4 November in the first year of his reign [1461], for the true and faithful allegiance and service which your said suppliant owed and did to the most blessed and Christian prince King Henry VI, your uncle, it was ordained and decreed that your same suppliant, by the name of William, Viscount Beaumont, should be unable henceforth to have, hold, inherit or enjoy any name of dignity, estate or pre-eminence within England, Ireland, Wales or Calais, or in their marches. And that your said suppliant and his heirs should be unable to claim or have any such name, estate or pre-eminence by him. And that your same suppliant, among others, should stand and be convicted of high treason, and forfeit to the said Edward late king and his heirs all the castles, manors, lands, lordships, tenements, rents, services, fees, advowsons, hereditaments and possessions, with their appurtenances, which he had by inheritance, or anyone else had to his use on 4 March in the said first year, or into which your same suppliant, or any other person or persons, feoffees to his use or benefit, had lawful cause of entry on the same 4 March, within England, Ireland, Wales or Calais, or in their marches, as is more fully contained in the same act May it please your highness, in consideration of the foregoing, by the advice and assent of the lords spiritual and temporal and of the commons assembled in this your present parliament, and by authority of the same, to ordain, decree and enact that the said act, and all acts of attainder and forfeiture made or had in the said parliament, or in any other parliament held in the time of the said Edward late king, against your said suppliant and his heirs, be void, annulled and of no force or effect against him and his heirs, and each of them. And that your said suppliant and his heirs be restored, enabled and have all such name, dignity, estate and pre-eminence, and also inherit, enter, have, hold and enjoy all the castles, lordships, manors, lands, tenements, reversions, services, advowsons and other possessions and hereditaments forfeited by the said act or acts, or by any of them, as well as by all others whatever they may be, in such manner and form, and in as large and valid a way as your same suppliant should or might have had or done if the said act or acts, or any of them, had never been had or made; notwithstanding the same acts, or any of them. And that the same act or acts, or any of them, or any letters patent made by occasion or reason of them, shall not be harmful or prejudicial in any way to your said suppliant or to his heirs, or to any feoffee or feoffees to his use at any time, concerning the things stated, or any part of them, but be entirely void against them, and each of them; and that he and his heirs, and all feoffees to the use of him or of his heirs, and of each of them, may have such advantage in everything, and be in as good a case and condition as if the said act or acts, or any of them, had never been had or made. And that nobody who, before the first day of this present parliament, has taken any issues or profits of the aforesaid castles, lordships, manors, lands, tenements or other things stated, or of any part of them, or intervened in them to the use or by the commandment of the said Edward late king, or of Richard III late in deed and not by right king of

England, or by virtue or means of any letters patent made by either of them to any person, shall be sued, vexed or troubled in any way for taking any such profits or intervening before the same first day by your said suppliant, or any of his heirs or executors, or by any of them, or by any other feoffee to the use of your said suppliant at any time, or any of them, but be entirely quit and discharged of the same against them, and each of them, by the aforesaid authority; saving to each of the king's liege people such right, title and interest in, of and to the things stated, and every part of them, as they or any of them had in the same things stated, or any part of them, when the same act was made or at any time since, other than by occasion of the same act or by any letters patent made or had by reason of the same act.

7. The Act of Parliament declaring William, Viscount Beaumont, unfit to take care of his possessions, November 1487:

Where William, Viscount Beaumont, in the time of King Edward IV, by authority of parliament was attainted of high treason by an act of attainder, and by the same forfeited to the same late king all his inheritance, of which our sovereign lord the king was seised on the strength of the same act from the beginning of the reign of our sovereign lord until our said sovereign lord, trusting that the same viscount was of good and serious disposition and rule, and had the discretion to rule himself and his livelihood to his honour and profit, without alienation or doing anything to disinherit himself or his heirs, had the same act of attainder reversed and the same viscount restored to his name and estate as well as to his said inheritance. Since that restoration our said sovereign lord has become convinced that the same viscount does not have the gravity and discretion to rule and keep himself or his said livelihood, but since that time has alienated, wasted, spoiled and put away a great part of it most unwisely, to the disinheritance of him and his heirs, and in all likelihood, should he have his liberty, he would hereafter deal with what is left in the same way.

In consideration of which, and since our said sovereign lord is bound to make provision for such persons as have inheritance and lack the gravity and discretion to rule and keep the same without alienation or the disinheritance of their heirs, by the advice of the lords spiritual and temporal and the commons assembled in this present parliament, and by authority of the same, be it ordained, decreed and enacted that our sovereign lord the king, or such as his grace shall depute, shall have the rule, disposition and guidance of all the livelihood and inheritance to which the said viscount was restored by the act of restitution made for him in the parliament held in the first year of the reign of our said sovereign lord, during the life of the same viscount, to the honour, maintenance and profit of the said viscount; and that the same viscount, during that time, shall have no authority or power to give or grant any part of it to any person without the assent or agreement of our said sovereign lord, while the said viscount is in the custody of our said sovereign lord, or the assent and agreement of such as his grace shall depute to have the rule of the said livelihood and inheritance; saving to all the king's liege people, other than the said viscount, such right, title and lawful interest as they have in or to any of the things stated.

8. The Act of Parliament declaring William, Viscount Beaumont, unfit to take care of himself, October 1495

Item, another bill concerning the custody of the Viscount Beaumont and his possessions and hereditaments was presented to the said king in the aforesaid parliament by the aforesaid commons, together with the tenors of certain provisos appended to the said bill, as will appear in what now follows:

Where in the parliament held at Westminster on 9 November in the third year of the reign of our sovereign lord the king [1487], it was ordained, decreed and enacted, for various good considerations contained in the said act, that our said sovereign lord or such as his grace should depute should have the rule, disposition and guidance of all the livelihood and inheritance of William, Viscount Beaumont, to which the said viscount was restored by an act of restitution made for him in the parliament held at Westminster in the first year of our said sovereign lord's reign [1485], during the life of the said viscount; and that the said viscount during that time should have no authority to give or grant any part of it to any person without the assent and agreement of our said sovereign lord or the assent and agreement of such as his grace should depute, while the said viscount was in the keeping of our said sovereign lord, or of such as his grace should depute to have the rule of the said livelihood or inheritance; in which act it was not clear what form the king's licence should take in that matter, or how the person of the said viscount should be kept, ordered, guided and conducted, but it was left open, as a result of which things might be done which were not to the king's honour, or to the worship of this land, considering he is a person descended of the noble blood of this land. For which reason it is ordained, enacted and decreed by authority of this present parliament that the king our sovereign lord, or such as he has or shall depute and assign, shall take and have the conduct, rule, keeping and governance, during the life of the [col. b] said viscount, of the person of the said viscount as well as of his said livelihood and inheritance, to be applied to the sustenance and maintenance of the said viscount as well as to the payment of his debts and otherwise, as shall be thought necessary and desirable by the king our sovereign lord, and by such as he has or shall depute and assign in that matter; and that the said viscount shall have no authority or power to give, grant, charge or alienate any part of his said livelihood or inheritance during his said life without the king's licence under his great seal; and if any alienation, gift, grant or charge has been made by him without obtaining the king's licence under his great seal in that matter since the said act was made in the said third year of his reign, except presentations to churches, chapels and chantries, then that alienation, gift, grant or charge shall stand and be entirely void and of no effect, except for those before excepted: and that no person shall hereafter be vexed or hurt by the said viscount, his executors or any other person claiming to his use any part of the said livelihood or inheritance, for any occupation or intervention, by reason of this act or since the said act made in the said third year of the king our sovereign lord's reign.

9. Elizabeth Scrope, Countess of Oxford's will, in which there is a sharp contrast between her mentions of her first husband, William Beaumont, Viscount Beaumont, and her second husband, John de Vere, Earl of Oxford:

http://www.oxford-shakespeare.com/Probate/PROB_11-27_ff_84-6.pdf.

RM: Tes[tamen]tu[m] D[omine] Elizabeth[e] Comitisse Oxon[ie] [f. 84r] In dei No[m]i[n]e Amen. I, Elizabeth, Countess of Oxenford, being in my pure widowhood and in my perfect mind and memory, knowing and considering the mutable and uncertain state of this present life, desiring to be in readiness whensoever it shall please our most merciful Saviour to call me from the same, do ordain and make this my present testament and last will the 30th day of May in the year of our Lord God 1537 and in the 29th year of the reign of our Sovereign Lord King Henry the 8th in manner and form following, that is to say:

First, I give and bequeath my soul unto the infinite mercy of Almighty God, Maker and Redeemer of the same, to the most blessed and glorious Virgin, Our Lady Saint Mary, and to all the holy company of heaven, and my body to be buried in the parish church of Wivenhoe by the corps and body of my dear Lord and sometime husband William, late Viscount Beaumont, whose soul Jesus pardon, utterly renouncing all manner of pomp and vain expenses in and about the same, and I renounce and revoke by this my testament and last will all other former testaments, wills, bequests and legacies by me made afore the date above-written; I will that all my debts sufficiently proved to be due by any writing or otherwise by me owing to any person be wholly and truly contented and paid, and in like manner I will that unto all persons duly and sufficiently proving that I have injured or wronged them, or taken any goods of them against reason and good conscience, be made full recompense and restitution, and forasmuch as I have had experience that to general doles as well the rich as the poor and needy persons do resort, I will therefore that no such common doles be made for me if mine executors by any good means may by their wisdom otherwise use it, and that I will to every parish near adjoining to the place of my burial be delivered by mine executors to the curate or curates, the churchwardens, & certain other honest men of every of the said parishes, such sums of money as shall be thought by mine executors convenient towards the relief of the poor and impotent persons of every of the said parishes, [RM: And in the church of every of the said parishes] I desire to have upon the thirty day next after my departure from this present life or thereabouts Dirge and Mass of Requiem to be said or sung, for the which to be done I will the curate, clerk or clerks of every of the said parishes to have competent reward by the discretion of mine executors, at which Mass and Dirge I will and desire that all and every poor people within their own parish to be present there to pray for my soul, my father, my mother, my husband's souls, and all Christian souls except he or they have a reasonable cause to be absent;

Also I will in like manner certain sums of money to be distributed by the discretion of my executors to the curates, clerks and poor people of every parish and parishes, as well where I am patroness as where I have lands and livelihood, for like intent and purpose as afore is mentioned;

Item, I will and require mine executors that they, as shortly after my decease as they may or convenient[ly] can provide, shall cause to be said or sung for my soul, for the souls of my father and mother, and my Lord my husband's soul, two hundred Masses, that is to say, fifty of the Trinity, fifty of the Holy Ghost, fifty of the Five Wounds, and fifty of Requies, and to reward the sayers of the said Masses for every Mass so often times said or sung, 12d in money;

Item, I give and bequeath to the picture of Our Blessed Lady of Walsingham, in th' honour of God and her, my marrying ring, or else the value of the same ring to be distribute amongst the poor people dwelling within the same town of Walsingham; this I defer unto the discretion of my executors;

Item, I give & bequeath to the parish church of Wivenhoe my best vestment and my best cope of crimson velvet, my best chalice, and my 2 altar-cloths of crimson velvet with a pane of blue velvet in the midst of the same, and a frontlet of the same suit; Also I give and bequeath to the chantry there, for the altar of Saint John the Baptist within the same church, 2 altar- cloths of blue velvet with a pane of crimson velvet in the midst of them, and one frontlet of white cloth of baudekin and crimson paned; Also, I give and bequeath to the abbess of Barking and to her sisters 4 marks in money, they to sing Dirge and Mass of Requies for my soul and the souls afore-named; Also I give and bequeath to the high altar of the church of Syon besides London my best altar-cloth of white cloth of baudekin, and to the brethren and sisters there being four marks in money for like intent afore rehearsed; to the brethren of the Charterhouse of Sheen for like [f. 84v] intent, 40s in money; to the brethren of the Charterhouse in London for like intent, other 40s in money; to the Nunnery Minors in London for like intent, other 40s in money; to the abbess and nuns of Denny for like intent, four marks in money; I give and bequeath to Dame Ursula Brewes, my niece, to pray for my soul, 40s in money; to the Friars Preachers in Cambridge for Dirge and Mass to be sung there for the souls afore-named, four nobles in money; to the Grey Friars in Colchester for like intent,

20s in money; to the Crossed Friars in Colchester for like intent, 10s in money; to the Friars Augustines of Clare for like intent, 20s in money; to the Friars Preachers in Sudbury for like intent, other 20s in money; to the Friars Preachers in London for Dirge and Mass for my soul and my father there buried, 40s in money; and to the Friars Augustines in Norwich for Dirge and Mass for my soul & mother there buried, 40s in money; Also I give and bequeath to 3 scholars of Cambridge to pray for my soul and the souls afore-named, to every of them four marks in money for one time; Also I give and bequeath to the chantry of Donington in Suffolk one of my copes of blue cloth of baudekin;

Item, I give and bequeath to the poor prisoners in Colchester Castle, in Newgate within London, in the Marshalsea and in the King's Bench in Southwark, in Melton jail in Suffolk, in the Castle of Cambridge, in Hertford jail, and in the shire jails of Lincoln and Leicester, to either of the said jails in ready money 6s 8d, to be distribute amongst the poor prisoners there;

Item, I give and bequeath to the right honourable and my singular good Lord, John de Vere, now Earl of Oxenford, 7 tapets of counterfeit arras of the story of Solomon lately by me bought of the Bishop of Ely['s] executors;

Item, a round sparver of yellow and russet satin [LM: paned, embroidered with roses & letters of gold & curtains of yellow & russet sarsenet] to the same;

Item, a tester of tinsel satin and black velvet paned for a trussing bed, embroidered with clouds and drops of gold, and four curtains of purple sarsenet to the same, and a trussing bedstead belonging to the same tester lately by me bought of the Lady Curson;

Item, 2 of my best featherbeds with 2 bolsters, 2 long pillows, 2 pair of fustians, 2 pair of sheets of 3 breadths, 2 long pillow-beres fine;

Item, 2 counterpoints, one of them of counterfeit arras with the picture of Saint George, lately bought of the said Lady Curson, and the other of (blank);

Item, I give and bequeath unto my said Lord my long cushion and 2 short cushions, the one side of them of needlework with silk, and the other side of incarnation satin embroidered with the Garter and letters of cloth of gold;

Item, my pax of silver and gilt, and a little box of silver to put in the Sacrament of the Altar;

Item, my great shaving-basin of silver weighing 80 ounces, and for a special remembrance, my little cross of gold having closed in the same a piece of the Holy Cross, which I daily wear about my neck;

Item, I give and bequeath to my Lord Bulbeck, my godson, my ring of gold with a rose of diamonds, & to the Lady Dorothy, his wife, a tablet of gold fastened like a steeple, set with divers small pearls and three blue stones with a pearl in the midst of them;

Item, I give and bequeath to his brother, Aubrey, my godson, my ring of gold with a sapphire of divers squares;

Item, I give and bequeath to the Lady Surrey, his sister, a book of gold having divers leaves of gold with the Salutation of Our Lady at the beginning; Item, to my god-daughter, Elizabeth Darcy, his sister, my ring largest with a sharp diamond; Item, to the Lady Anne Vere, his sister, a book of gold of the value of 100s with the picture of the Crucifix and the Salutation of Our Lady, to be newly made;

Item, I give and bequeath to my god-daughter, Elizabeth Howard, a tablet of gold with th' Assumption of Our Lady and Saint Francis;

Item, I give and bequeath to my sister Vere my image of Our Lady of Pity, to hang at her beads to pray for my soul; Item, to my niece Wingfield, her daughter, my ring with the Five Joys of Our Lady with a table diamond;

Item, I give and bequeath to my brother, Sir William Kingston, knight, my Jesus of diamonds set in gold with 3 great pearls hanging at the same, also my 2 flagons of silver having my Lord of Oxenford's arms in them;

Item, I give and bequeath to my sister, Dame Mary, his wife, a basin and an ewer of silver chased gilt of the newest making afore the chance of fire, weighing 92 ounces; my goblet of gold graven with crankettes and mullets, weighing 13 ounces 1 quarter; and also my book of gold set with pearl;

Item, I give and bequeath to my sister, Jane Brewes, a basin and an ewer chased gilt of the oldest sort, weighing five score and 6 ounces, having my Lord of Oxenford['s] arms in the bottom of the basin; Item, a great goblet with the cover of silver, parcel-gilt, weighing 31 ounces, graven with crankettes and mullets, which she lately gave me after the chance of fire;

Item, my cross of gold ragged which was my father's, accustomably worn about my neck;

Item, a trussing bed of black velvet and scarlet cloth engrained paned, embroidered with letters of cloth of gold and black velvet, a counterpoint of the same, one featherbed with a bolster, 2 pillows, 2 pair of sheets of 2 breadths di[medium], and one pair of fustians;

Item, I give and bequeath to my sister, Dame Mary Kingston, and to my sister, Jane Brewes, all my samplers, evenly to be divided between them, and I will my said sister Kingston to have the choice;

Item, I give and bequeath unto my brother [=brother-in-law], Sir John Seyntclere, knight, a basin and an ewer of silver chased gilt, the fellow of the same that I have bequeathed unto my sister Brewes, weighing five score and 6 ounces;

Item, I give and bequeath unto my sister [=half-sister], Dame Frances, his wife, a cup of silver and gilt of the value of £4 sterling, or else £4 in ready money; Item, my trussing bed of black velvet and black satin paned, with curtains of tawny sarsenet to the same;

Item, a counterpoint of blue cloth of baudekin, one featherbed with bolster, one long pillow, one pair of fustians, and 2 pair of sheets of 2 breadths and a half;

Item, I give and bequeath unto Dame Alice Cotton, widow, my beads of black jet large gauded with crosses of gold;

Item, I give and bequeath unto Philip Paris, esquire, my basin and an ewer of silver parcel-gilt, weighing 78 ounces, and if the said basin be not of the whole value of £20 sterling, that then I will he shall have so much money as the said basin and ewer lacketh of the value of £20;

Item, I give and bequeath unto my nephew, Henry Jerningham, my great balas standing in gold with a white rose and a red enameled, and 3 pearls hanging at the same; also, I give and bequeath him ten pounds sterling;

Item, I give and bequeath my nephew, John Brewes, my cross of gold with the Five Wounds and a flower-de-luce of diamonds;

Item, I give and bequeath unto my nephew, John Seyntclere, one of my great goblets of silver all gilt with a cover to the same, having a grayle of flower-de-luce about the same goblet;

Item, I give and bequeath unto my nephew, Edmund Jerningham, a goblet of silver and gilt with a cover, weighing 15 ounces di[medium], the goblet pounced like pens, having my Lord Beaumont's arms and mine in the top of the cover, and also I give him fifty pounds in ready money;

Item, I give and bequeath to my niece Luttrell my tablet of gold pictured with the Crucifix, Our Lady, and Saint John;

Item, I give and bequeath unto my niece Audley a standing cup of silver and gilt with a cover, newly made, weighing 30 ounces di[medium], di[medium] quarter;

Item, I give and bequeath to my nephew, John Wyndham, a round hoop of gold with a small pointed diamond;

Item, I give and bequeath to my nephew, Giles Brewes, a standing cup of silver and gilt with a cover, newly made, weighing 24 ounces di[medium], di[medium] quarter;

Item, I give & bequeath to John Beaumont, esquire, my goblets of silver and gilt with a cover, weighing together 45 ounces 3 quarters di[medium], and also five pounds in ready money;

Item, I give and bequeath to my nephew, Giles Seyntclere, my godson, a cross of gold with the Crucifix and the letters of I.N.R.I;

Item, I give and bequeath to John Danyell, my receiver, a standing cup of silver and gilt with a cover, newly made, weighing 37 ounces di[medium], di[medium] quarter, to be of the value of £10 sterling;

Item, I give and bequeath to my niece, Elizabeth Seyntclere, one of my beer-pots of silver and gilt; Item, a gown of black satin, a kirtle of black velvet, and also towards the advancement of her marriage I give her threescore pounds in ready money which her father, Sir John Seyntclere, knight, is indebted unto me, as appeareth by divers bills of his handwriting remaining in my hands and custody, and over and besides that I give and bequeath her forty pounds in money to be delivered by mine executors;

Item, I give & bequeath to my cousin, Dame Margaret Scrope, five pounds in money;

Item, I give and bequeath to Muriel Christmas my ring with a diamond like a spear-point;

Item, I give and bequeath to Jane Crane my ring with a turquoise;

Item, I give and bequeath to Ely Fyncham my ring with an emerald;

Item, I give and bequeath unto Elizabeth Rve my pomander of gold like a pear, used to be worn at my girdle; Item, I give and bequeath to Elizabeth Miche a pair of Eyeleres(?) beads gauded with 10 beads of gold; Item, I give and bequeath to my nephew, Edmund Audley, a cup of silver and gilt with the cover, of the value of five pounds in money;

Item, I give and bequeath to Anthony Stapleton, towards his learning at the common law, ten pounds in money;

Item, I give and bequeath to Margaret Ryther th' elder, for the true and faithful service that she of long continuance hath done to me, one hundred marks in ready money, 2 salts of silver and gilt with a cover and a Garter in the midst of them, weighing 26 ounces; Item, 2 of my best featherbeds not before bequeathed; Item, 4 pair of my best sheets, 2 bolsters, 2 pillows, one long, and 2 mattresses, 2 counterpoints, the one having the pictures of Saint John the Baptist, Saint Peter and Saint Giles of counterfeit arras, used to be laid upon my bed, the other like unto the same of counterfeit arras; Item, 2 pair of fustians; Item, all my tappets of tapestry of damask-work, the ground green, with the Garter and my Lord's arms in them, used to be hanged in my chamber;

Item, 2 brass pots of 3 gallons, 2 small pans of brass, and one garnish of counterfeit vessel largest of pewter;

Item, I give and bequeath to John Ryther, my controller of household, 2 pots of silver parcel-gilt which I lately bought of Master Lucas, weighing 64 ounces one quarter, and also 2 bowls of silver parcel-gilt of the value of £11 6s 8d, and for lack of the same bowls, he to have of my gift £11 6s 8d in ready money; Item, I give and bequeath to Margaret, his wife, my trussing bed of blue velvet and crimson, my counterpoint of yellow Turkey satin and curtain of yellow sarsenet to the same; Item, 2 featherbeds, 2 bolsters, 2 pillows, 2 pillow-beres, 2 pair of sheets and one pair of fustians;

Item, I give to my god-daughter, Elizabeth Ryther, five pounds in ready money, and to John Ryther, her brother, other five pounds in ready money;

Item, I give and bequeath to Robert Goldingham, my gentleman-usher, for his continuant good service, ten pounds in ready money; Item, I give and bequeath to John Fabyan, marshal of my hall, for his good faithful service, twenty nobles in money;

Item, I give and bequeath to Doctor Cranker, my almoner, my 2 salts of silver and gilt with one cover, having a scripture about them, weighing 45 ounces one quarter;

Item, I give and bequeath to Mr Robert Skinner, my chaplain, five pounds in ready money;

Item, I give and bequeath to Master Ralph Bane, my chaplain, other five pounds in ready money;

Item, I give and bequeath to Elizabeth Bowes, one of my maidens, for her long service, twenty pounds in money;

Item, I give and bequeath to Elizabeth Willoughby, for her good service, twenty marks in ready money;

Item, to Margaret Frognall for like cause, 20 marks in ready money;

Item, to Jane Roberts, for like cause, 20 marks in ready money;

Item, to Ele Fyncham, for like cause, 20 nobles in ready money;

Item, I give and bequeath to Emlyn Badbye, my chamberer, for her good service, 20 marks in ready money;

Item, I give and bequeath unto my said 6 women all mine apparel except my jewels and gowns of velvet and satin, equally divided among them by the discretion of my executors;

Item, I give and bequeath to Frances Baynham, one of my maidens, five pounds in ready money;

Item, I give and bequeath to Katherine Christmas, one of my maidens, a pair of beads of crystal gauded with beads of gold;

Item, I give and bequeath to Mary Hamersham, towards the advancement of her marriage, ten marks in ready money;

Item, I give and bequeath to Christopher Goldingham my trussing bed of crewel needlework with roses and a counterpoint of silk dornick;

Item, one featherbed, one bolster, 2 pillows, one pair of sheets, and one pair of fustians;

Item, I give to Anne, his wife, one long cushion and 2 short cushions of crewel of damask-work with the needle, and my small pair of beads of jet gauded with beads of gold;

Item, I give and bequeath to John Goldingham, his son, five pounds in ready money; to Robert Rochester, gentleman, for his good service unto me done, ten marks in ready money;

Item, I give and bequeath to Richard Hardekyn, yeoman usher of my chamber, for his old continuant service to me done, five pounds in ready money, one featherbed, one bolster, and one coverlet of white tapestry with the letters of E and O;

Item, I will that every chaplain and gentleman waiter being in my checker-roll not before remembered in this my will with any special bequest shall have one featherbed, one bolster, one pair of sheets and one coverlet shortly after my departure;

Item, I will that all such my servants as shall be in my checker-roll at my departure shall incontinent after my said departure have their whole year's wages over and besides any legacies or bequests to any of them by this my present testament and last will given;

Item, I will that all other my servants as retained, not being in my checker-roll, shall have incontinent after my departure their yearly remembrance which they had in my lifetime for one time;

Item, I give and bequeath to old Trott and his wife, or the longest liver of them, 20s in ready money, and also one bed with th' appurtenances at the discretion of my executors;

Item, I will that all my featherbeds, sheets, fustians, counterpoints and all other stuff of household before in this my present testament and last will given and bequeathed and not declared or assigned by name nor by special token be delivered at the discretion of my executors;

Item, I will that all my plate, jewels, my stuff of household and all other my moveable goods not given nor bequeathed in this my last will and testament be sold by mine executors to the best proof that may conveniently be for the performance of this my said last will and testament, and that fulfilled, I will the overplus be disposed and distribute as well amongst my most needy and poor servants as in other deeds of charity by the discretion of mine executors for the weal of my soul, my father and mother's souls, my Lords' and husbands' soul[s], and all Christian souls;

Item, I will that every of mine executors taking upon him the charges of execution of this my present testament and last will shall have ten pounds in ready money for his pains taking in and about the same;

Also I will that all and every of my said executors so taking the charge upon them shall have all such charges and costs as shall be sustained by any of them in any manner of wise in and about th' execution of this my present testament and last will; Also I give and bequeath to Sir Thomas Cromwell, Lord Cromwell and Lord Privy Seal, for a poor remembrance, ten pounds in ready money, desiring and willing him to be supervisor of this my present testament and last will;

And for the performance of this my present testament and last will I ordain and make mine executors whose names are hereafter with mine own hand written; In witness whereof I have set to my sign manual in the presence of them that hereafter unto this my will hath set to their hands bearing witness that this is my last will and testament: my brother Sir William Kingston, knight; Philip Paris, squire; my sister, Jane [sic] Kingston; Margaret Rider, and John Ryder. By me, Elizabeth Oxenford.

10. A Victorian opinion on mediaeval mental health care: Henry Alfred Napier, in the book *Historical Notices of the Parishes of Swyncombe and Ewelme in the County of Oxfordshire*, 1863:

The charities of the middle ages were perhaps not more redundant or more misapplied than those of our own day, and many of them were eminently beneficial. There were hospitals for the sick and infirm, lying-in hospitals, asylums for the aged, the impotent, and the insane. Bedlam existed then, and was devoted to the same purposes as at present. And, whatever may have been the system of treatment adopted for the patients, it appears that some were cured; and the charity of the age extended a large indulgence to all who were so afflicted.

Endnotes

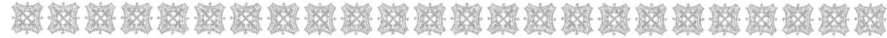

Preface

1. Professor Mark Williams, *Cry of Pain. Understanding Suicide and the Suicidal Mind.* (London: Little, Brown Book Group, 2014) p.3.
2. Ibid.

Introduction

3. Ralph Alan Griffiths, *The Reign of Henry VI. The Exercise of Royal Authority.* (Berkeley: University of California Press, 1981) p.175.
4. Ibid.

Chapter 1: Famous cases

5. For example detailed in: Thomas F. Graham, *Medieval Minds: Mental Health in the Middle Ages.* (London: Taylor & Francis, 2019) 'Bartholomew'.
6. Tig Lang, 'Medical Recipes from the Yorkist Court' in *The Ricardian*, June 2010, pp.94–102.
7. Ibid.
8. Warren R. Dawson, *A Leecbboole or Collection of Medical Recipes of the Fifteenth Century.* (London, 1934) pp.299–300.

9. K.B. McFarlane, *England in the Fifteenth Century*. (London: Bloomsbury Academic, 1981) p.42.
10. Ibid.
11. Keith Dockray, *Henry VI, Margaret of Anjou and the Wars of the Roses. From Contemporary Chronicles, Letters & Records*. (Stroud: Fonthill Media, 2016) p.22.
12. Bertram Wolffe, *Henry VI*. (London: Yale University Press, 2001) position 6182.
13. Ibid., pp.5–14.
14. Ibid., position 7875.
15. For example: Lauren Johnson, *Shadow King: The Life and Death of Henry VI*. (London: Head of Zeus Ltd, 2019) pp.150/1.
16. For example: Matthew Lewis, *Richard, Duke of York: King by Right*. (Stroud: Amberley Publishing, 2016) p.372.
17. Ibid.
18. Keith Dockray, *Henry VI, Margaret of Anjou and the Wars of the Roses. From Contemporary Chronicles, Letters & Records*. (Stroud: Fonthill Media, 2016) p.10.
19. Lauren Johnson: *Shadow King. The Life and Death of Henry VI*. (London: Head of Zeus Ltd, 2019) p.301 ff.
20. Ibid.
21. Keith Dockray, *Henry VI, Margaret of Anjou and the Wars of the Roses. From Contemporary Chronicles, Letters & Records*. (Stroud: Fonthill Media, 2016) pp.48–53.
22. Matthew Lewis, *Richard, Duke of York: King by Right*. (Stroud: Amberley Publishing, 2016) p.313.
23. Ibid.
24. Lauren Johnson, *Shadow King. The Life and Death of Henry VI*. (London: Head of Zeus Ltd, 2019) p.472.
25. For example: Bertram Wolffe, *Henry VI*. (London: Yale University Press, 2001) positions 7210–7227.
26. Keith Dockray, *Henry VI, Margaret of Anjou and the Wars of the Roses. From Contemporary Chronicles, Letters & Records*. (Stroud: Fonthill Media, 2016) pp.50–1.
27. Matthew Lewis, *Richard, Duke of York: King by Right*. (Stroud: Amberley Publishing, 2016) p.232.
28. John Silvester Davies (ed.), *An English chronicle of the reigns of Richard II, Henry IV, Henry V, and Henry VI written before*

the year 1471; with an appendix, containing the 18th and 19th years of Richard II and the Parliament at Bury St. Edmund's, 25th Henry VI and supplementary additions from the Cotton. ms. chronicle called 'Eulogium'. (London: Camden Society, 1856) pp.94–96.
29. Robert Bale, *De Præfectis et Consulibus Londini*. 1461.
30. 'Henry VII: November 1487', in *Parliament Rolls of Medieval England*, (eds.) Chris Given-Wilson, Paul Brand, Seymour Phillips, Mark Ormrod, Geoffrey Martin, Anne Curry and Rosemary Horrox (Woodbridge, 2005), *British History Online:* http://www.british-history.ac.uk/no-series/parliament-rolls-medieval/november-1487.
31. As explained in: Alexander Murray, *Suicide in the Middle Ages: The violent against themselves*. (Oxford: Oxford University Press, 1998) pp.55–58.
32. James Ross, *The Foremost Man of the Kingdom. John de Vere, Thirteenth Earl of Oxford (1442–1513)*. (Woodbridge: Boydell Press, 2011) p.82.
33. Ibid.
34. 'Henry VII: October 1495', in *Parliament Rolls of Medieval England*, (eds). Chris Given-Wilson, Paul Brand, Seymour Phillips, Mark Ormrod, Geoffrey Martin, Anne Curry and Rosemary Horrox (Woodbridge, 2005), *British History Online:* http://www.british-history.ac.uk/no-series/parliament-rolls-medieval/october-1495.
35. James Ross, *The Foremost Man of the Kingdom. John de Vere, Thirteenth Earl of Oxford (1442–1513)*. (Woodbridge: Boydell Press, 2011) p.82.
36. Ibid., pp.96–7.
37. Ibid., p.97.
38. Ibid.
39. Lakshmi, N., Yatham, Mario Maj, *Bipolar Disorder. Clinical and Neurobiological Foundations*. (New York: John Wiley and Sons, 2011.)
40. Ibid.
41. Stefan Zweig, *Friedrich Nietzsche - Der Tanz über dem Abgrund. Eine Biografie*. (Leipzig, Insel-Verlag, 1925) pp.10–11.
42. http://www.oxford-shakespeare.com/Probate/PROB_11-27_ff_84-6.pdf.

43. Claire Trenery, *Peregrine Horden, Madness in the Middle Ages*, in: Ed. Greg Eghigan, *The Routledge History of Madness and Mental Health* (London: Routledge, 2017) pp.66–7.
44. J. L. Laynesmith, *Cecily, Duchess of York*. (London, New York: Bloomsbury Academic, 2017) pp.62–79.
45. Calendar of Patent Rolls, Henry VI, Volume IV, AD 1446–1452, p.430.
46. K. L. Clark, *The Nevills of Middleham: England's Most Powerful Family in the Wars of the Roses*. (Stroud: The History Press, 2016) p.228.
47. John Burke, *A General and Heraldic Dictionary of the Peerages of England, Ireland, and Scotland, Extinct, Dormant, and in Abeyance*. (London: H. Colburn & R. Bentley, 1831) pp.301–2.
48. Ibid., p.392.
49. 'Gregory's Chronicle: 1461–1469', in *The Historical Collections of a Citizen of London in the Fifteenth Century*, (ed.) James Gairdner (London, 1876), pp.210–239. *British History Online:* http://www.british-history.ac.uk/camden-record-soc/vol17/pp.210–239.
50. Ibid.
51. K. L. Clark, *The Nevills of Middleham: England's Most Powerful Family in the Wars of the Roses*. (Stroud: The History Press, 2016) p.308.
52. Ibid., p.228.
53. 'Henry VI: November 1450', in *Parliament Rolls of Medieval England*, (eds.) Chris Given-Wilson, Paul Brand, Seymour Phillips, Mark Ormrod, Geoffrey Martin, Anne Curry and Rosemary Horrox (Woodbridge, 2005), *British History Online:* http://www.british-history.ac.uk/no-series/parliament-rolls-medieval/november-1450.
54. Ibid.
55. Ibid.
56. The battle is detailed in: Ian Mortimer: *1415: Henry V's Year of Glory*. (London: Random House, 2009) pp.388–464.
57. Ibid.
58. Ibid.
59. Helmut Feld, *Jeanne d'Arc: geschichtliche und virtuelle Existenz des Mädchens von Orleans*. (Münster: LIT, 2016) p.271.

60. Ibid., p.37.
61. Ian Mortimer, *1415: Henry V's Year of Glory.* (London: Random House, 2009) p.517.
62. Lauren Johnson, *Shadow King. The Life and Death of Henry VI.* (London: Head of Zeus Ltd, 2019) p.102.
63. Ibid., p.103.
64. Keith Dockray, *Henry VI, Margaret of Anjou and the Wars of the Roses. From Contemporary Chronicles, Letters & Records.* (Stroud: Fonthill Media, 2016) p.44.
65. Susan Curran, *The English Friend.* (Norwich: Lasse Press, 2011.) position 1718.
66. See: Keith Dockray, *Henry VI, Margaret of Anjou and the Wars of the Roses. From Contemporary Chronicles, Letters & Records.* (Stroud: Fonthill Media, 2016) pp.48–50.
67. *Chronique du Religieux de Saint-Denys, contenant le règne de Charles VI, de 1380 à 1422, publiée en latin pour la première fois et traduite par M. Louis-François Bellaguet, précédée d'une introduction de M. de Barante.* (Paris: Crapelet, 1839–1852) pp.19–23.
68. Thomas Basin and Charles Samaran (eds.), *Histoire de Charles VII: Tome Premier, 1407–1444.* (Paris: Les Classiques de l'Histoire de France Au Moyen Age. Volume 15, 1933) pp.394–5.
69. *Chronique du Religieux de Saint-Denys, contenant le règne de Charles VI, de 1380 à 1422, publiée en latin pour la première fois et traduite par M. Louis-François Bellaguet, précédée d'une introduction de M. de Barante.* (Paris: Crapelet, 1839–1852) pp.19–23.
70. Ibid.
71. Ibid.
72. Keith Dockray, *Henry VI, Margaret of Anjou and the Wars of the Roses. From Contemporary Chronicles, Letters & Records.* (Stroud: Fonthill Media, 2016) pp.49–50.
73. Thomas Basin and Charles Samaran (eds.), *Histoire de Charles VII: Tome Premier, 1407–1444.* (Paris: Les Classiques de l'Histoire de France Au Moyen Age. Volume 15, 1933) pp.394–5.
74. Ibid.
75. https://www.newadvent.org/cathen/12297a.htm.
76. Ibid.

77. *Chronique du Religieux de Saint-Denys, contenant le règne de Charles VI, de 1380 à 1422, publiée en latin pour la première fois et traduite par M. Louis-François Bellaguet, précédée d'une introduction de M. de Barante.* (Paris: Crapelet, 1839–1852) pp.19–23.
78. Salvatore Poeta, 'The Hispanic and Luso-Brazilian World: From Mad Queen to Martyred Saint: The Case of Juana La Loca Revisited in History and Art on the Occasion of the 450th Anniversary of Her Death' in *Hispania* Vol. 90, No. 1 (March 2007) pp.165–172 (8 pages). Published By: American Association of Teachers of Spanish and Portuguese.
79. Ibid.
80. Ibid.
81. Professor Bethany Aram, *Juana the Mad. Sovereignty and Dynasty in Renaissance Europe.* (Baltimore: Johns Hopkins University Press, 2008) pp.108, 201.
82. Ibid.
83. Ibid.
84. Dixie Dennis, *Living, Dying, Grieving.* (Sudbury: Jones & Bartlett Learning, 2008) p.148.
85. Professor Bethany Aram, *Juana 'the Mad's' Signature: The Problem of Invoking Royal Authority, 1505–1507*, p.332.
86. Lauren Johnson, *Shadow King: The Life and Death of Henry VI.* (London: Head of Zeus Ltd, 2019) p.498.
87. Ibid., pp.498–502.
88. Professor Bethany Aram, *Juana 'the Mad's' Signature: The Problem of Invoking Royal Authority, 1505–1507*, p.332.
89. Ibid.
90. Ibid.
91. Ibid.
92. James Gairdner, *The Paston Letters, AD 1422–1509. Volume VI.* New Complete Library Edition (London: Chatto & Windus, Exeter: James G. Commin, 1904) pp.1–3.
93. Ibid.
94. N. Denholm-Young, Wendy R. Childs (eds.), *Vita Edwardi Secundi.* (Oxford: Clarendon Press, 2005) p.22.
95. 'Lateran Regesta 43: 1396–1397', in *Calendar of Papal Registers Relating To Great Britain and Ireland: Volume 4, 1362–1404,*

W. H. Bliss and J. A. Twemlow (eds.) (London, 1902), pp.542–546. *British History Online* http://www.british-history.ac.uk/cal-papal-registers/brit-ie/vol4/pp542–546.
96. Nicola Tallis, *Uncrowned Queen: The Fateful Life of Margaret Beaufort, Tudor Matriarch.* (London: Michael O'Mara Books Limited, 2019) position 734.
97. For example: Lauren Johnson, *Shadow King: The Life and Death of Henry VI.* (London: Head of Zeus Ltd, 2019) p.206.
98. H. T. Riley, *Ingulph's Chronicle of the Abbey of Croyland.* (London: George Bell and Sons, 1908) p.399.
99. Ibid.
100. Lauren Johnson, *Shadow King: The Life and Death of Henry VI.* (London: Head of Zeus Ltd, 2019) p.194.
101. H. T. Riley, *Ingulph's Chronicle of the Abbey of Croyland.* (London: George Bell and Sons, 1908) p.399.
102. Ibid.
103. Nicola Tallis, *Uncrowned Queen: The Fateful Life of Margaret Beaufort, Tudor Matriarch.* (London: Michael O'Mara Books Limited, 2019) p.729.
104. As explained in: Claire Trenery, 'Peregrine Horden, Madness in the Middle Ages' in Greg Eghigan (ed.), *The Routledge History of Madness and Mental Health.* (London: Routledge, 2017) pp.66–7.
105. John Bruce (ed.), *Historie of the Arrivall of Edward IV in England and the Finall Recouerye of his Kingdomes from Henry VI AD M.CCCC.LXXI.* (London: John Bower Nichols and Son, 1838) p.38.
106. J. Halliwell (ed.), *A Chronicle of the First Thirteen Years of the Reign of Edward IV by John Warkworth.* (London: 1839) p.20.
107. See, for example: Reginald Robinson Sharpe, *Calendar of coroners rolls of the city of London, A.D. 1300–1378.* (London: R. Clay & Sons, 1913) and by H. E. Salter (ed.), *Records of mediaeval Oxford. Coroners' inquests, the walls of Oxford.*
108. Ibid.
109. Catharine Arnold, *Bedlam. London and Its Mad.* (London: Simon & Schuster, 2009) p.3.
110. Alexander Murray, *Suicide in the Middle Ages: The violent against themselves.* (Oxford: Oxford University Press, 1998) p.111.
111. Ibid.

112. Ibid.
113. Ibid.
114. Ibid.
115. Reginald Robinson Sharpe, *Calendar of coroners rolls of the city of London, A.D. 1300–1378.* (London: R. Clay & Sons, 1913) p.96.
116. Ibid.
117. For example: H. E. Salter (ed.), *Records of mediaeval Oxford. Coroners' inquests, the walls of Oxford.*
118. Alexander Murray, *Suicide in the Middle Ages: The violent against themselves.* (Oxford: Oxford University Press, 1998) p.3.

Chapter 2: Treatments for mental illnesses

119. Great Britain. Privy Council, Nicholas Harris Nicolas, and Great Britain. Record Commission. *Proceedings And Ordinances of the Privy Council of England ...* (London: Printed by G. Eyre and A. Spottiswoode), 183437.
120. Lauren Johnson, *Shadow King. The Life and Death of Henry VI.* (London: Head of Zeus Ltd, 2019).
121. Great Britain. Privy Council, Nicholas Harris Nicolas, and Great Britain. Record Commission. *Proceedings And Ordinances of the Privy Council of England ...* (London: Printed by G. Eyre and A. Spottiswoode), 183437.
122. Ibid.
123. *Cry of Pain. Understanding Suicide and the Suicidal Mind.* (London: Little, Brown Book Group, 2014) p.14.
124. Lauren Johnson, *Shadow King. The Life and Death of Henry VI.* (London: Head of Zeus Ltd, 2019) p.303.
125. Charles Teo, Michael E. Sughrue, *Principles and Practice of Keyhole Brain Surgery.* (Stuttgart, New Delhi, New York, Rio: George Thieme Verlag, 2015).
126. Catharine Arnold, *Bedlam. London and Its Mad.* (London: Simon & Schuster, 2009) p.72.
127. Ibid.
128. Ibid., p.133.
129. Ibid., pp.138, 169.

130. Ibid., pp.3, 133.
131. Ibid.
132. Peter Laurie (LL. B.), *A narrative of the proceedings at the laying of the first stone of the new buildings at Bethlem hospital.* (London: Governors of Bridewell and Bethlem Hospitals, 1838) p.40.
133. Ibid.
134. Catharine Arnold, *Bedlam. London and Its Mad.* (London: Simon & Schuster, 2009) pp.62, 63.
135. Ibid., p.6.
136. Ibid., p.3.
137. See, for example: Alexander Murray, *Suicide in the Middle Ages: The violent against themselves.* (Oxford: Oxford University Press, 1998) pp.12, 13.
138. Ibid.
139. Ibid., p.111.
140. Claire Trenery, 'Peregrine Horden, Madness in the Middle Ages' in Greg Eghigan (ed.), *The Routledge History of Madness and Mental Health.* (London: Routledge, 2017) pp.66–7.
141. Ibid.
142. Ibid.
143. Ibid.
144. Ibid.
145. Ibid.
146. Ibid.
147. Catharine Arnold, *Bedlam. London and Its Mad.* (London: Simon & Schuster, 2009) pp.28, 67, 207.
148. Claire Trenery, 'Peregrine Horden, Madness in the Middle Ages' in: Greg Eghigan (ed.), *The Routledge History of Madness and Mental Health.* (London: Routledge, 2017) pp.66–7.
149. For example: Angela Dailey, *Cooking to Cure. A Nutritional Approach to Anxiety and Depression.* (CreateSpace Independent Publisher, 2015).
150. Catharine Arnold, *Bedlam. London and Its Mad.* (London: Simon & Schuster, 2009) p.36.
151. Claire Trenery, 'Peregrine Horden, Madness in the Middle Ages' in Greg Eghigan (ed.), *The Routledge History of Madness and Mental Health.* (London: Routledge, 2017) pp.66–7.

152. Ibid.
153. Ibid.
154. Ibid.
155. Catharine Arnold, *Bedlam. London and Its Mad.* (London: Simon & Schuster, 2009) p.6.
156. Ibid., p.201.
157. Ibid.
158. Ibid.
159. Ibid.
160. Ibid., pp.65, 66.
161. https://www.rethink.org/advice-and-information/living-with-mental-illness/treatment-and-support/.
162. Keith Dockray, *Henry VI, Margaret of Anjou and the Wars of the Roses. From Contemporary Chronicles, Letters & Records.* (Stroud: Fonthill Media, 2016) pp.49–51.
163. Claire Trenery, 'Peregrine Horden, Madness in the Middle Ages' in Greg Eghigan (ed.), *The Routledge History of Madness and Mental Health.* (London: Routledge, 2017) pp.66–7.
164. Ibid.
165. Ibid.
166. Greg Eghigan (ed.), *The Routledge History of Madness and Mental Health.* (London: Routledge, 2017) pp.66–7.
167. Catharine Arnold, *Bedlam. London and Its Mad.* (London: Simon & Schuster, 2009) pp.65, 66.
168. Ibid., p.221.
169. Greg Eghigan (ed.), *The Routledge History of Madness and Mental Health.* (London: Routledge, 2017) pp.62–64.
170. Ibid.
171. Monika H. Green, *The Trotula: A Medieval Compendium of Women's Medicine.* (The Middle Ages Series) (Philadelphia: University of Pennsylvania Press, 2001) 5 percent.
172. Ibid.
173. Ibid.
174. Ibid.
175. Ibid.
176. Ibid.
177. Ibid.
178. Ibid.

179. Catharine Arnold, *Bedlam. London and Its Mad.* (London: Simon & Schuster, 2009) p.10.
180. https://www.rethink.org/advice-and-information/living-with-mental-illness/treatment-and-support/.
181. Donna Trembinski, *Illness and Authority. Disability in the Life and Lives of Francis of Assisi.* (Toronto: University of Toronto Press, 2020) p.131.
182. For example: Ibid., p.115.
183. Ibid., p.10, 71.
184. Ibid., p.71
185. https://www.british-history.ac.uk/search/series/cal-papal-registers--brit-ie.
186. Ibid.
187. Ibid.
188. Donna Trembinski, *Illness and Authority. Disability in the Life and Lives of Francis of Assisi.* (Toronto: University of Toronto Press, 2020) p.114.
189. Ibid., p.10, 71.
190. Ibid., p.53.
191. Ibid., p.127.
192. Ibid.
193. Helen Castor, *Joan of Arc. A history.* (London: Faber and Faber Ltd, 2014).
194. For example, Ibid.; also: Helmut Feld, *Jeanne d'Arc: geschichtliche und virtuelle Existenz des Mädchens von Orleans.* (Münster: LIT, 2016.)
195. Ibid., pp.30, 39.
196. Ibid.
197. Ibid.
198. Ibid., p.251.
199. See. Raphael Holinshed, *Chronicles of England, Scotland and Ireland* (1577).
200. Greg Eghigan (ed.), *The Routledge History of Madness and Mental Health.* (London: Routledge, 2017) pp.62–64.
201. Ibid.
202. Ibid.
203. Ibid.
204. Ibid.

205. Ibid.
206. Claire Trenery, 'Peregrine Horden, Madness in the Middle Ages' in Greg Eghigan (ed.), *The Routledge History of Madness and Mental Health*. (London: Routledge, 2017) pp.66–7.
207. Ibid.
208. Ibid.
209. Ibid.
210. Catharine Arnold, *Bedlam. London and Its Mad*. (London: Simon & Schuster, 2009) p.130.
211. Claire Trenery, 'Peregrine Horden, Madness in the Middle Ages' in Greg Eghigan (ed.), *The Routledge History of Madness and Mental Health*. (London: Routledge, 2017) pp.66–7.
212. Susan Wise Bauer, *The History of the Renaissance World: From the Rediscovery of Aristotle to the Conquest of Constantinople*. (New York: W. W. Norton & Company, 2013) p.46.
213. Ibid.
214. Thomas Penn, *Winter King: Henry VII and the Dawn of Tudor England*. (London: Penguin Books Ltd, 2011.)
215. Ibid.
216. Ibid.
217. For example: John Ashdown-Hill, *The Third Plantagenet*. (Stroud: The History Press, 2014.)
218. Thomas Penn, *Winter King: Henry VII and the Dawn of Tudor England*. (London: Penguin Books Ltd, 2011.)
219. James D. Taylor, *The Shadow of the White Rose. Edward Courtenay, Earl of Devon, 1526–1556*. (New York: Algora Publishing, 2006.)
220. Ibid.
221. Ibid.
222. Ibid.
223. Catharine Arnold, *Bedlam. London and Its Mad*. (London: Simon & Schuster, 2009) p.307.
224. As referenced in, for example: Alexander Murray, *Suicide in the Middle Ages: The violent against themselves*. (Oxford: Oxford University Press, 1998) pp.251–294.
225. Nicholas Orme, *Medieval Children*. (New Haven and London: Yale University Press, 2001.)
226. Ibid.
227. Ibid.

228. Ibid.
229. Ibid.
230. Ibid.
231. Ibid.
232. Ibid.
233. Ibid.
234. Ibid.
235. Ibid.

Chapter 3: Societal reaction

236. 'Henry VII: November 1487', in *Parliament Rolls of Medieval England*, (eds). Chris Given-Wilson, Paul Brand, Seymour Phillips, Mark Ormrod, Geoffrey Martin, Anne Curry and Rosemary Horrox (Woodbridge, 2005), *British History Online:* http://www.british-history.ac.uk/no-series/parliament-rolls-medieval/november-1487 and 'Henry VII: October 1495', in *Parliament Rolls of Medieval England*, (eds.) Chris Given-Wilson, Paul Brand, Seymour Phillips, Mark Ormrod, Geoffrey Martin, Anne Curry and Rosemary Horrox (Woodbridge, 2005), *British History Online* http://www.british-history.ac.uk/no-series/parliament-rolls-medieval/october-1495.
237. Robert Bale, *De Præfectis et Consulibus Londini*. 1461.
238. Ibid.
239. Keith Dockray, *Henry VI, Margaret of Anjou and the Wars of the Roses. From Contemporary Chronicles, Letters & Records.* (Stroud: Fonthill Media, 2016) p.49.
240. Ibid.
241. Ibid., p.50.
242. For example: Thomas Basin and Charles Samaran (eds.), *Histoire de Charles VII: Tome Premier, 1407–1444*. (Paris: Les Classiques de l'Histoire de France Au Moyen Age. Volume 15, 1933.)
243. Lauren Johnson, *Shadow King. The Life and Death of Henry VI*. (London: Head of Zeus Ltd, 2019) p.301.
244. Ibid., p.302.
245. Ibid., p.301.
246. Ibid., pp.301–2.
247. Ibid.

248. Ibid.
249. An example is given: Ibid., p.391.
250. Ibid.
251. Thomas Basin and Charles Samaran (eds.), *Histoire de Charles VII: Tome Premier, 1407–1444*. (Paris: Les Classiques de l'Histoire de France Au Moyen Age. Volume 15, 1933.)
252. Lauren Johnson, *Shadow King. The Life and Death of Henry VI.* (London: Head of Zeus Ltd, 2019) p.302.
253. Keith Dockray, *Henry VI, Margaret of Anjou and the Wars of the Roses. From Contemporary Chronicles, Letters & Records.* (Stroud: Fonthill Media, 2016) pp.48–50.
254. Nicholas Orme, *Medieval Children.* (New Haven and London: Yale University Press, 2001.)
255. Ibid.
256. Ibid.
257. Ibid.
258. Ibid.
259. Keith Dockray, *Henry VI, Margaret of Anjou and the Wars of the Roses. From Contemporary Chronicles, Letters & Records.* (Stroud: Fonthill Media, 2016) pp.48–51.
260. Lauren Johnson, *Shadow King. The Life and Death of Henry VI.* (London: Head of Zeus Ltd, 2019) pp.30–34.
261. Ibid. p.112; Matthew Lewis, *Richard, Duke of York: King by Right.* (Stroud: Amberley Publishing, 2016) pp.105–6.
262. Keith Dockray, *Henry VI, Margaret of Anjou and the Wars of the Roses. From Contemporary Chronicles, Letters & Records.* (Stroud: Fonthill Media, 2016) p.50.
263. Ibid., pp.48–51.
264. https://d.lib.rochester.edu/teams/publication/simpson-pevereley-hardyng-chronicle.
265. Thomas F. Graham, *Medieval Minds: Mental Health in the Middle Ages.* (London: Taylor & Francis, 2019) 'Bartholomew'.
266. Reginald Robinson Sharpe, *Calendar of coroners rolls of the city of London, A.D. 1300–1378.* (London: R. Clay & Sons, 1913.)
267. Ibid.
268. Ibid.
269. Ibid.
270. Ibid.

271. Ibid.
272. Thomas F. Graham, *Medieval Minds: Mental Health in the Middle Ages*. (London: Taylor & Francis, 2019) 'Bartholomew'.
273. Reginald Robinson Sharpe, *Calendar of coroners rolls of the city of London, A.D. 1300–1378*. (London: R. Clay & Sons, 1913.)
274. Salvatore Poeta, 'The Hispanic and Luso-Brazilian World: From Mad Queen to Martyred Saint: The Case of Juana La Loca Revisited in History and Art on the Occasion of the 450th Anniversary of Her Death' in *Hispania* Vol. 90, No. 1 (March 2007), pp.165–172 (8 pages). Published By: American Association of Teachers of Spanish and Portuguese.
275. Mary Clive, *This Son of York. A biography of Edward IV*. (London: Macmillan London Ltd, 1973) p.84.
276. Ibid.
277. Ibid.
278. 'Henry VI: March 1453', in *Parliament Rolls of Medieval England*, (eds.) Chris Given-Wilson, Paul Brand, Seymour Phillips, Mark Ormrod, Geoffrey Martin, Anne Curry and Rosemary Horrox (Woodbridge, 2005). *British History Online:* http://www.british-history.ac.uk/no-series/parliament-rolls-medieval/march-1453.
279. Thomas Penn, *Winter King: Henry VII and the Dawn of Tudor England*. (London: Penguin Books Ltd, 2011) p.112.
280. Ibid.
281. 'Henry VI: March 1453', in *Parliament Rolls of Medieval England*, (eds.) Chris Given-Wilson, Paul Brand, Seymour Phillips, Mark Ormrod, Geoffrey Martin, Anne Curry and Rosemary Horrox (Woodbridge, 2005). *British History Online:* http://www.british-history.ac.uk/no-series/parliament-rolls-medieval/march-1453.
282. Ibid.
283. Ibid.
284. Bertram Wolffe, *Henry VI*. (London: Yale University Press, 2001) p.6515.
285. Ibid., position 6660.
286. Matthew Lewis, *Richard, Duke of York: King by Right*. (Stroud: Amberley Publishing, 2016) p.372.
287. Ibid.
288. 'Henry VI: March 1453', in *Parliament Rolls of Medieval England*, (eds). Chris Given-Wilson, Paul Brand, Seymour

Phillips, Mark Ormrod, Geoffrey Martin, Anne Curry and Rosemary Horrox (Woodbridge, 2005). *British History Online:* http://www.british-history.ac.uk/no-series/parliament-rolls-medieval/march-1453.
289. Matthew Lewis, *Richard, Duke of York: King by Right*. (Stroud: Amberley Publishing, 2016) p.372.
290. Great Britain. Privy Council, Nicholas Harris Nicolas, and Great Britain. Record Commission. *Proceedings And Ordinances of the Privy Council of England* ... [London: Printed by G. Eyre and A. Spottiswoode], 183437.
291. Greg Eghigan (ed.), *The Routledge History of Madness and Mental Health*. (London: Routledge, 2017) pp.66–7.
292. 'Henry VI: March 1453', in *Parliament Rolls of Medieval England*, (eds). Chris Given-Wilson, Paul Brand, Seymour Phillips, Mark Ormrod, Geoffrey Martin, Anne Curry and Rosemary Horrox (Woodbridge, 2005). *British History Online:* http://www.british-history.ac.uk/no-series/parliament-rolls-medieval/march-1453.
293. Bertram Wolffe, *Henry VI*. (London: Yale University Press, 2001) position 6660.
294. Lauren Johnson, *Shadow King. The Life and Death of Henry VI*. (London: Head of Zeus Ltd, 2019) p.305 ff.
295. Ibid.
296. 'Henry VI: March 1453', in *Parliament Rolls of Medieval England*, (eds.) Chris Given-Wilson, Paul Brand, Seymour Phillips, Mark Ormrod, Geoffrey Martin, Anne Curry and Rosemary Horrox (Woodbridge, 2005). *British History Online:* http://www.british-history.ac.uk/no-series/parliament-rolls-medieval/march-1453.
297. Keith Dockray, *Henry VI, Margaret of Anjou and the Wars of the Roses. From Contemporary Chronicles, Letters & Records*. (Stroud: Fonthill Media, 2016) pp.45–51.
298. Matthew Lewis, *Richard, Duke of York: King by Right*. (Stroud: Amberley Publishing, 2016) pp.328.
299. John Silvester Davies (ed.), *An English chronicle of the reigns of Richard II, Henry IV, Henry V, and Henry VI written before the year 1471; with an appendix, containing the 18th and 19th years of Richard II and the Parliament at Bury St. Edmund's, 25th Henry VI and supplementary additions from the Cotton. ms. chronicle called 'Eulogium'*. (London: Camden Society, 1856.)

300. *REGISTRUM ABBATIÆ JOHANNIS WHETHAMSTEDE, ABBATIS MONASTERII SANCTI ALBANI, ITERUM SUSCEPTÆ.* Published online by Cambridge University Press: 05 August 2013.
301. 'Henry VI: November 1449', in *Parliament Rolls of Medieval England*, (eds.) Chris Given-Wilson, Paul Brand, Seymour Phillips, Mark Ormrod, Geoffrey Martin, Anne Curry and Rosemary Horrox (Woodbridge, 2005). *British History Online.* http://www.british-history.ac.uk/no-series/parliament-rolls-medieval/november-1449.
302. Ibid.
303. Keith Dockray, *Henry VI, Margaret of Anjou and the Wars of the Roses. From Contemporary Chronicles, Letters & Records.* (Stroud: Fonthill Media, 2016) p.49.
304. Ibid., pp.45–51.
305. 'Henry VI: November 1449', in *Parliament Rolls of Medieval England*, (eds.) Chris Given-Wilson, Paul Brand, Seymour Phillips, Mark Ormrod, Geoffrey Martin, Anne Curry and Rosemary Horrox (Woodbridge, 2005). *British History Online.* http://www.british-history.ac.uk/no-series/parliament-rolls-medieval/november-1449.
306. Lauren Johnson, *Shadow King. The Life and Death of Henry VI.* (London: Head of Zeus Ltd, 2019) pp.253–264.
307. Matthew Lewis, *Richard, Duke of York: King by Right.* (Stroud: Amberley Publishing, 2016) p.182.
308. Lauren Johnson, *Shadow King: The Life and Death of Henry VI.* (London: Head of Zeus Ltd, 2019) pp.253–264.
309. Ibid.
310. Matthew Lewis, *Richard, Duke of York: King by Right.* (Stroud: Amberley Publishing, 2016) p.231.
311. Keith Dockray, *Henry VI, Margaret of Anjou and the Wars of the Roses. From Contemporary Chronicles, Letters & Records.* (Stroud: Fonthill Media, 2016) pp.48–51.
312. Matthew Lewis, *Richard, Duke of York: King by Right.* (Stroud: Amberley Publishing, 2016) p.140, 218–232.
313. Ibid.
314. Keith Dockray, *Henry VI, Margaret of Anjou and the Wars of the Roses. From Contemporary Chronicles, Letters & Records.* (Stroud: Fonthill Media, 2016) p.50.

315. Ibid.
316. Stanley Krippner, Daniel B. Pitchford, Jeannine Davies, *Post-traumatic Stress Disorder*. (Westport: Greenwood Publishing Group, 2012) p.21.
317. Keith Dockray, *Henry VI, Margaret of Anjou and the Wars of the Roses. From Contemporary Chronicles, Letters & Records.* (Stroud: Fonthill Media, 2016) p.49.
318. Ibid., pp.45–51.
319. Ibid.
320. For example: Bertram Wolffe, *Henry VI.* (London: Yale University Press, 2001) position 7862.
321. Lauren Johnson, *Shadow King. The Life and Death of Henry VI.* (London: Head of Zeus Ltd, 2019) p.150; and Ralph Alan Griffiths, *The Reign of Henry VI. The Exercise of Royal Authority.* (Berkeley: University of California Press, 1981.)
322. Matthew Lewis, *Richard, Duke of York: King by Right.* (Stroud: Amberley Publishing, 2016) p.285.
323. Keith Dockray, *Henry VI, Margaret of Anjou and the Wars of the Roses. From Contemporary Chronicles, Letters & Records.* (Stroud: Fonthill Media, 2016) pp.49–51.
324. Lauren Johnson, *Shadow King. The Life and Death of Henry VI.* (London: Head of Zeus Ltd, 2019) p.150; and Ralph Alan Griffiths, *The Reign of Henry VI. The Exercise of Royal Authority.* (Berkeley: University of California Press, 1981.)
325. For example: Bertram Wolffe, *Henry VI.* (London: Yale University Press, 2001) position 6919.
326. https://twitter.com/thehistoryguy/status/938517167229882368.
327. Keith Dockray, *Henry VI, Margaret of Anjou and the Wars of the Roses. From Contemporary Chronicles, Letters & Records.* (Stroud: Fonthill Media, 2016) pp.45–51.
328. Mary Clive: *This Son of York. A biography of Edward IV.* (London: Macmillan London Ltd, 1973) p.274.
329. Susan Curran, *The English Friend.* (Norwich: Lasse Press, 2011) position 2053.
330. Ibid., position 2024.
331. For example: 'Henry VI: March 1453', in *Parliament Rolls of Medieval England*, (eds.) Chris Given-Wilson, Paul Brand, Seymour Phillips, Mark Ormrod, Geoffrey Martin, Anne Curry

and Rosemary Horrox (Woodbridge, 2005). *British History Online.* http://www.british-history.ac.uk/no-series/parliament-rolls-medieval/march-1453.
332. As explained in: Thomas F. Graham, *Medieval Minds: Mental Health in the Middle Ages.* (London: Taylor & Francis, 2019).
333. Reginald Robinson Sharpe, *Calendar of coroners rolls of the city of London, A.D. 1300–1378.* (London: R. Clay & Sons, 1913.)
334. Thomas Basin and Charles Samaran (eds.), *Histoire de Charles VII: Tome Premier, 1407–1444.* (Paris: Les Classiques de l'Histoire de France Au Moyen Age. Volume 15, 1933).
335. Great Britain. Privy Council, Nicholas Harris Nicolas, and Great Britain. Record Commission. *Proceedings And Ordinances of the Privy Council of England* ... [London: Printed by G. Eyre and A. Spottiswoode], 183437.
336. Ibid.
337. Ibid.
338. Matthew Lewis, *Richard, Duke of York: King by Right.* (Stroud: Amberley Publishing, 2016) p.234.
339. Ibid., p.247.
340. Ibid.
341. Ibid.
342. Ibid.
343. Keith Dockray, *Henry VI, Margaret of Anjou and the Wars of the Roses. From Contemporary Chronicles, Letters & Records.* (Stroud: Fonthill Media, 2016) p.50.
344. Matthew Lewis, *Richard, Duke of York: King by Right.* (Stroud: Amberley Publishing, 2016) p.251.
345. Oliver, Clementine. 'Murdered in the Tabloids: Billposting and the Destruction of the Duke of Suffolk in 1450' in *Anales de la Universidad de Alicante. Historia Medieval, No. 19* (2015–2016): pp.381–402, DOI:10.14198/medieval.2015-2016.19.13.
346. Keith Dockray, *Henry VI, Margaret of Anjou and the Wars of the Roses. From Contemporary Chronicles, Letters & Records.* (Stroud: Fonthill Media, 2016) p.49.
347. Professor Bethany Aram, *Juana the Mad. Sovereignty and Dynasty in Renaissance Europe.* (Baltimore: Johns Hopkins University Press, 2008) p.152.
348. Ibid., p.109.

349. Ibid.
350. Ibid.
351. Ibid., p.88.
352. Salvatore Poeta, 'The Hispanic and Luso-Brazilian World: From Mad Queen to Martyred Saint: The Case of Juana La Loca Revisited in History and Art on the Occasion of the 450th Anniversary of Her Death' in *Hispania* Vol. 90, No. 1 (March 2007) pp.165–172 (8 pages). Published By: American Association of Teachers of Spanish and Portuguese.
353. Ibid.
354. Ibid.
355. Ibid.
356. Ibid.
357. Ibid.
358. Ibid.
359. Professor Bethany Aram, *Juana the Mad. Sovereignty and Dynasty in Renaissance Europe*. (Baltimore: Johns Hopkins University Press, 2008) p.123.
360. https://www.rethink.org/advice-and-information/living-with-mental-illness/treatment-and-support/recovery/.
361. Professor Bethany Aram, *Juana the Mad. Sovereignty and Dynasty in Renaissance Europe*. (Baltimore: Johns Hopkins University Press, 2008) p.131.
362. Ibid., p.122.
363. Ibid., p.88.
364. For example: Ibid., p.88 ff.
365. Ibid., p.122.
366. Ibid., p.109.
367. Salvatore Poeta, 'The Hispanic and Luso-Brazilian World: From Mad Queen to Martyred Saint: The Case of Juana La Loca Revisited in History and Art on the Occasion of the 450th Anniversary of Her Death' in *Hispania* Vol. 90, No. 1 (March 2007) pp.165–172 (8 pages.) Published By: American Association of Teachers of Spanish and Portuguese.
368. Professor Bethany Aram, *Juana the Mad. Sovereignty and Dynasty in Renaissance Europe*. (Baltimore: Johns Hopkins University Press, 2008) p.151ff.
369. Ibid.

370. Salvatore Poeta, 'The Hispanic and Luso-Brazilian World: From Mad Queen to Martyred Saint: The Case of Juana La Loca Revisited in History and Art on the Occasion of the 450th Anniversary of Her Death' in *Hispania* Vol. 90, No. 1 (March 2007) pp.165–172 (8 pages). Published By: American Association of Teachers of Spanish and Portuguese.
371. Ibid.
372. Professor Bethany Aram, *Juana the Mad. Sovereignty and Dynasty in Renaissance Europe.* (Baltimore: Johns Hopkins University Press, 2008) p.1.
373. See, for example, the mediaeval cures mentioned in: Thomas F. Graham, *Medieval Minds: Mental Health in the Middle Ages.* (London: Taylor & Francis, 2019.)
374. Salvatore Poeta, 'The Hispanic and Luso-Brazilian World: From Mad Queen to Martyred Saint: The Case of Juana La Loca Revisited in History and Art on the Occasion of the 450th Anniversary of Her Death' in *Hispania* Vol. 90, No. 1 (March 2007) pp.165–172 (8 pages). Published By: American Association of Teachers of Spanish and Portuguese.
375. Professor Bethany Aram, *Juana the Mad. Sovereignty and Dynasty in Renaissance Europe.* (Baltimore: Johns Hopkins University Press, 2008) p.108.
376. Ibid.
377. Greg Eghigan (ed.), *The Routledge History of Madness and Mental Health.* (London: Routledge, 2017) pp.62–67.
378. Ibid.
379. Ibid.
380. A. Okerlund, *Elizabeth of York.* (London: Palgrave Macmillan US, 2009) pp.209, 210.
381. Michèle Schindler, *Lovell Our Dogge. The Life of Viscount Lovell, Closest Friend of Richard III and Failed Regicide.* (Stroud: Amberley Publishing, 2019) pp.39, 40.
382. 'Henry VII: October 1495', in *Parliament Rolls of Medieval England*, (eds.) Chris Given-Wilson, Paul Brand, Seymour Phillips, Mark Ormrod, Geoffrey Martin, Anne Curry and Rosemary Horrox (Woodbridge, 2005). *British History Online.* http://www.british-history.ac.uk/no-series/parliament-rolls-medieval/october-1495.

383. Mentioned, for example, in: Thomas F. Graham, *Medieval Minds: Mental Health in the Middle Ages*. (London: Taylor & Francis, 2019.)
384. The religious ramifications of this, and especially the consequences if these witnesses were found lying: Ibid.
385. Ibid.
386. Ibid.
387. Charles Ross, *Edward IV*. (New Haven and London: Yale University Press, 1974.)
388. John Ashdown-Hill, *The Third Plantagenet*. (Stroud: The History Press, 2014.)
389. 'Edward IV: January 1478', in *Parliament Rolls of Medieval England*, (eds.) Chris Given-Wilson, Paul Brand, Seymour Phillips, Mark Ormrod, Geoffrey Martin, Anne Curry and Rosemary Horrox (Woodbridge, 2005). *British History Online:* http://www.british-history.ac.uk/no-series/parliament-rolls-medieval/january-1478.
390. Ibid.
391. George's entire story is found in: John Ashdown-Hill, *The Third Plantagenet*. (Stroud: The History Press, 2014.)
392. H. T. Riley, *Ingulph's Chronicle of the Abbey of Croyland*. (London: George Bell and Sons, 1908) pp.143–145.
393. John Ashdown-Hill, *The Third Plantagenet*. (Stroud: The History Press, 2014) p.149.
394. Ibid.
395. Charles Ross, *Edward IV*. (New Haven and London: Yale University Press, 1974.)
396. John Ashdown-Hill, *The Third Plantagenet*. (Stroud: The History Press, 2014.)
397. Ibid., pp. 132, 133.
398. 'Edward IV: January 1478', in *Parliament Rolls of Medieval England*, (eds.) Chris Given-Wilson, Paul Brand, Seymour Phillips, Mark Ormrod, Geoffrey Martin, Anne Curry and Rosemary Horrox (Woodbridge, 2005). *British History Online:* http://www.british-history.ac.uk/no-series/parliament-rolls-medieval/january-1478.
399. Ibid.
400. Matthew Lewis, *Richard III: Loyalty Binds Me*. (Stroud: Amberley Publishing, 2018.) position 6666.
401. For example: Lauren Johnson, *Shadow King: The Life and Death of Henry VI*. (London: Head of Zeus Ltd, 2019) p.150.

402. Bertram Wolffe, *Henry VI*. (London: Yale University Press, 2001) position 7862.
403. Ibid.
404. John Ashdown-Hill, *The Third Plantagenet*. (Stroud: The History Press, 2014) pp.132, 133
405. *Harleian Manuscripts* 433 Vol. 3, p.108.
406. Raphael Holinshed, *Chronicles of England, Scotland and Ireland*. (1577.)
407. John Ashdown-Hill, *The Third Plantagenet*. (Stroud: The History Press, 2014) pp.132, 133.
408. *Harleian Manuscripts* 433 Vol. 3, p.108.
409. Ibid.
410. As mentioned above, in: Thomas F. Graham, *Medieval Minds: Mental Health in the Middle Ages*. (London: Taylor & Francis, 2019.)
411. Ibid.

Chapter 4: Religion and mental illness

412. Ibid., p.65.
413. Ibid., pp.40, 41, 78.
414. Ibid., p. 65.
415. Ibid.
416. As discussed in: Helen Castor: *Joan of Arc: A History*. (London: Faber and Faber Ltd, 2014.)
417. Ibid.
418. Ibid.
419. Ibid.
420. Ibid.
421. Ibid.
422. Ibid.
423. Thomas Basin and Charles Samaran (eds.), *Histoire de Charles VII: Tome Premier, 1407–1444*. (Paris: Les Classiques de l'Histoire de France Au Moyen Age. Volume 15, 1933.)
424. Ibid.
425. Ibid.
426. Thomas F. Graham, *Medieval Minds: Mental Health in the Middle Ages*. (London: Taylor & Francis, 2019) pp. 40, 41, 78.

427. Ibid.
428. Ibid.
429. Greg Eghigan (ed.), *The Routledge History of Madness and Mental Health.* (London: Routledge, 2017) p.106.
430. Ibid., p.93
431. Ibid.
432. Ibid.
433. Ibid.
434. Ibid.
435. Ibid., p.65
436. Helen Castor, *Joan of Arc. A history.* (London: Faber and Faber Ltd, 2014.)
437. Greg Eghigan (ed.), *The Routledge History of Madness and Mental Health.* (London: Routledge, 2017) p.93.
438. Ibid.
439. Professor Bethany Aram, *Juana the Mad. Sovereignty and Dynasty in Renaissance Europe.* (Baltimore: Johns Hopkins University Press, 2008) p.20.
440. Robin R. Mundill, *The King's Jews: Money, Massacre and Exodus in Medieval England.* (London: Bloomsbury, 2010) p.154.
441. As can be seen in: *Records of the Spanish Inquisition. Translated from the Original Manuscripts.* (London: Samuel G. Goodrich, 1828.)
442. Professor Bethany Aram, *Juana the Mad. Sovereignty and Dynasty in Renaissance Europe.* (Baltimore: Johns Hopkins University Press, 2008) p.106.
443. Ibid.
444. Ibid.
445. Ibid.
446. Salvatore Poeta, *The Hispanic and Luso-Brazilian World: From Mad Queen to Martyred Saint: The Case of Juana La Loca Revisited in History and Art on the Occasion of the 450th Anniversary of Her Death*, Hispania Vol. 90, No. 1 (March 2007) pp.165–172 (8 pages) Published By: American Association of Teachers of Spanish and Portuguese
447. Ibid.
448. Professor Bethany Aram, *Juana the Mad. Sovereignty and Dynasty in Renaissance Europe* (Baltimore: Johns Hopkins University Press, 2008)

449. *Records of the Spanish Inquisition. Translated from the Original Manuscripts* (London: Samuel G. Goodrich, 1828)
450. Professor Bethany Aram, *Juana the Mad. Sovereignty and Dynasty in Renaissance Europe* (Baltimore: Johns Hopkins University Press, 2008) p.106.
451. Ibid.
452. Ibid.
453. Ibid.
454. As seen in: *Records of the Spanish Inquisition. Translated from the Original Manuscripts.* (London: Samuel G. Goodrich, 1828.)
455. Ibid.
456. Ibid.
457. Ibid.
458. Ibid.
459. Ibid.
460. Ibid.
461. Catharine Arnold, *Bedlam. London and Its Mad.* (London: Simon & Schuster, 2009) pp.28, 67, 207.
462. *Records of the Spanish Inquisition. Translated from the Original Manuscripts.* (London: Samuel G. Goodrich, 1828.)
463. Greg Eghigan (ed.), *The Routledge History of Madness and Mental Health.* (London: Routledge, 2017) p.93.
464. Ibid.
465. This is explained in Catharine Arnold, *Bedlam. London and Its Mad.* (London: Simon & Schuster, 2009) p.62.
466. Thomas F. Graham, *Medieval Minds: Mental Health in the Middle Ages.* (London: Taylor & Francis, 2019) pp. 22, 42, 86.
467. Ibid.
468. Ibid.
469. Ibid.
470. Ibid.
471. Ibid.
472. Dorinda Outram, *Panorama of the Enlightenment.* (Los Angeles: Getty Trust Publications, 2006) pp.201, 314.
473. Thomas F. Graham, *Medieval Minds: Mental Health in the Middle Ages.* (London: Taylor & Francis, 2019) pp.77, 78, 86.
474. Ibid.

475. As explained in: Greg Eghigan (ed.), *The Routledge History of Madness and Mental Health*. (London: Routledge, 2017.)
476. Ibid.
477. https://www.rethink.org/advice-and-information/living-with-mental-illness/treatment-and-support/recovery/.
478. P. Leese, *Traumatic Neurosis and the British Soldiers of the First World War.* (London: Palgrave Macmillan UK, 2002.)
479. Thomas F. Graham, *Medieval Minds: Mental Health in the Middle Ages*. (London: Taylor & Francis, 2019), for example p.102.
480. Greg Eghigan (ed.), *The Routledge History of Madness and Mental Health.* (London: Routledge, 2017) p.63.
481. Dorinda Outram, *Panorama of the Enlightenment.* (Los Angeles: Getty Trust Publications, 2006) pp. 201, 314.
482. As quoted: Ibid.
483. Ibid.
484. Greg Eghigan (ed.), *The Routledge History of Madness and Mental Health.* (London: Routledge, 2017) p.63.
485. Ibid.
486. Fiona Maddocks, *Hildegart of Bingen. The Woman of her Age.* (Leipzig: Faber & Faber, 2013) 'Physician and Healer'.
487. Ibid., 'Visions'.
488. Ibid.
489. Ibid., 'Papal Approval'.
490. Ibid.
491. Ibid., 'Correspondence and Friendship'.
492. Ibid.
493. Ibid., 'Visions'.
494. Ibid.
495. Ibid.
496. https://www.rethink.org/advice-and-information/living-with-mental-illness/treatment-and-support/recovery/
497. Fiona Maddocks, *Hildegart of Bingen. The Woman of her Age.* (Leipzig: Faber & Faber, 2013) 'Papal Approval'.
498. Günther H. Heepen, *Das Heilwissen der Hildegard von Bingen. Naturheilmittel – Ernährung – Edelsteine.* (München: Gräfe und Unzer Verlag GmbH, 2015), for example: p.21.
499. Ibid.

500. Fiona Maddocks, *Hildegart of Bingen. The Woman of her Age.* (Leipzig: Faber & Faber, 2013) 'Visions'.
501. Günther H. Heepen, *Das Heilwissen der Hildegard von Bingen. Naturheilmittel – Ernährung – Edelsteine* (München: Gräfe und Unzer Verlag GmbH, 2015).
502. Fiona Maddocks, *Hildegart of Bingen. The Woman of her Age.* (Leipzig: Faber & Faber, 2013) 'Visions', 'Papal Approval'.
503. Ibid.
504. Ibid.
505. Ibid., 'Relighting the Flame', 'Shrines and Icons'.
506. As explained: Ibid., 'Childhood and Cloister'.
507. Günther H. Heepen, *Das Heilwissen der Hildegard von Bingen. Naturheilmittel – Ernährung – Edelsteine* (München: Gräfe und Unzer Verlag GmbH, 2015) p.21.

Chapter 5: Mental health and mental illness in mediaeval literature

508. David Wright (ed.). Geoffrey Chaucer, *The Canterbury Tales.* (Oxford: Oxford University Press, 1998) p.83.
509. Ibid., p.90.
510. Ibid.
511. Ibid.
512. Ibid., p.99.
513. Ibid., p.83.
514. Ibid., p.99.
515. Ibid.
516. Ibid., pp.x–xxiv.
517. Ibid.
518. Ibid.
519. Some theories as to Chaucer and what he might have intended are found in: Marion Turner, *Chaucer: A European Life.* (Princeton and Oxford: Princeton University Press, 2019.)
520. Sir Thomas Malory, *Le Morte D'Arthur.* (London: Random House Publishing Group, 2000.)
521. A. Okerlund, *Elizabeth of York.* (London: Palgrave Macmillan US, 2009), p.39.

522. Sir Thomas Malory, *Le Morte D'Arthur.* (London: Random House Publishing Group, 2000) pp.449–493.
523. Ibid.
524. Ibid.
525. Terence H. White, *The Once and Future King.* (Roermond: Fontana, 1987.)
526. Sir Thomas Malory, *Le Morte D'Arthur.* (London: Random House Publishing Group, 2000) p.541.
527. Ibid., pp.449–493.
528. Ibid.